Healthy Nuts

Healthy Nuts

GENE SPILLER, PhD

AVERY PUBLISHING GROUP

Garden City Park • New York

The information contained in this book is based upon the research and the personal and professional experiences of the author. As the sole purpose of this book is to educate, every effort has been made to provide the most complete, current, and accurate information as possible. It is not intended as a substitute for consulting with your physician or other health-care provider. The publisher and author are not responsible for any adverse effects or consequences resulting from the use of any of the suggestions discussed in this book. All matters pertaining to your physical health should be supervised by a health-care professional. It is a sign of wisdom, not cowardice to seek a second or third opinion.

Cover designer: Phaedra Mastrocola
Cover photo credit: Jenni Haas Design
In-house editor: Dara Stewart
Typesetter: Gary A. Rosenberg
Illustrations: John Richards
Printer: Paragon Press, Honesdale, PA

Avery Publishing Group
120 Old Broadway
Garden City Park, NY 11040
1–800–548–5757
www.averypublishing.com

The Upside-Down Pyramid on page 113 is used courtesy of the Sphera Foundation.

Publisher's Cataloging-in-Publication Data

Spiller, Gene A.
    Healthy nuts : your guide to the healthful
  benefits of nuts / Gene Spiller. — 1st ed.
    p. cm.
    Includes bibliographical references and index.
    ISBN: 1-58333-011-9

    1. Nuts. 2. Nuts—Therapeutic use.
  I. Title.

SB401.A4S65 1999   641.3'45
                                     QBI99-1417

Printed in the United States of America

10   9   8   7   6   5   4   3   2   1

Contents

To my wife Monica,
whose love for real food
has inspired me for many years.

Acknowledgments

This book would not have been possible without the extensive material supplied to me by the International Tree Nut Council, headquartered in Reus, Spain, and by the various nut agricultural organizations. Special thanks go to Penny Kris-Etherton, Ph.D., Professor of Nutrition at Pennsylvania State University and a leading researcher in nut nutrition, whose collection of data, advice, and publications on nuts have been extremely helpful in the writing of this book.

Many scientists, physicians, and researchers have contributed original interviews, which have helped to add the opinions of leading researchers to this book. Thank you to Jeffrey B. Blumberg, Ph.D., Associate Director/Senior Scientist and Chief of the Antioxidants Research Laboratory; T. Colin Campbell, Ph.D., Professor of Nutritional Biochemistry and project director of the China-Oxford-Cornell Diet and Health Project at Cornell University in Ithaca, New York; John W. Farquhar, M.D., Professor of Medicine at Stanford University School of Medicine, Director of the Stanford University Wellness Center and Founder of the Center for Research in Disease Prevention; Gary E. Fraser, M.D., Ph.D., Professor of Medicine and Epidemiology at Loma Linda University and director of the Center for Health Research, School of Public Health in Loma Linda, California; David J.A. Jenkins, M.D., Ph.D., Professor of Medicine in the Departments of Medicine and Nutritional

Sciences at the University of Toronto and Director of the Risk Factor Modification Center at St. Michael's Hospital in Toronto; Larry Kushi, D.Sc., Associate Professor, Division of Epidemiology, School of Public Health at the University of Minnesota in Minneapolis; Jean Mayer of the USDA Human Nutrition Research Center on Aging at Tufts University in Boston, Massachusetts, and Professor in the School of Nutrition Science and Policy at Tufts University; Bandaru Reddy, D.V.M., Ph.D., Associate Professor, Chief of the Division of Nutritional Carcinogenesis at the American Health Foundation in Valhalla, New York; Gabriele Riccardi, M.D., Associate Professor of Metabolic Diseases and Chairman of Applied Dietetics at Federico II University Medical School in Naples, Italy; Joan Sabaté, M.D., Dr.P.H., Associate Professor of Nutrition, Epidemiology, and Biostatistics at Loma Linda University, Loma Linda, California; Rosemary Stanton, B.Sc., C.Nut., nutritionist in the Department of Medicine, University of New South Wales in Sydney, Australia; Antonia Trichopoulou, M.D., Professor of Nutrition and Biochemistry at the Athens School of Public Health, and Chief of the World Health Organization, Collaborating Center for Nutrition in Athens, Greece; and Walter C. Willett, Dr.P.H., M.D., Professor of Epidemiology and Nutrition and Chair of the Department of Nutrition at the Harvard School of Public Health in Boston, Massachusetts.

Not less important, several cookbook authors and chefs have helped with ideas either directly or through their publications. I must thank Monica Spiller, author of the *Barm Bakers' Book* and researcher of ancient foods; Jesse Cool, cookbook author and chef-owner of the Flea Street Café near Stanford University; Paula Wolfert, author of many books on Mediterranean cooking; and Deborah Madison, author and chef, who has contributed recipes to some of my previous books.

Many books have been invaluable sources of information, but some deserve special mention: Edwin Menninger's *Edible Nuts of the World*; *Indian Givers* by Jack Weatherford; *The Complete Book of Fruits and Vegetables* by Francesco Bianchini and co-authors; *To the King's Taste* by Lorna Sass; Constance Hieatt and Sharon Butler brought back medieval recipes in their *Curye on Inglysch: English Culinary Manuscripts of the Fourteenth Century*; Mary Reed's *Fruits*

& Nuts in Symbolism & Celebration; Heinerman's Encyclopedia of Nuts, Berries and Seeds by John Heinerman; and that always inspiring book on the history of food that is very dear to my heart, Reay Tannahill's *Food in History*.

John Richards, a Menlo Park, California, artist, created beautiful illustrations of each nut, and Rosemary Schmele has been invaluable in her assistance in the preparation of this manuscript.

And, finally, I want to thank Georgia Hughes, my literary agent, and my editor, Dara Stewart, at Avery Publishing, who helped to put the final touches on the manuscript.

Foreword

While nuts have numerous health benefits, they have not been recognized as being important to nutrition due to lack of awareness of these benefits. Consumption of a moderate amount of different types of nuts can help prevent chronic disease, including coronary heart disease and various kinds of cancer. As we move toward a balanced plant-based diet, the decrease in protein intake that occurs when one leaves behind animal products can be more than adequately compensated for by the excellent quality of protein present in nuts. This balance that nuts can provide is one of the great advantages of adding nuts to a plant-based diet. The protein in nuts is a high-quality mixture of amino acids, which can complement those obtained from other foods. There is some evidence that plant protein, in and of itself, can lower blood cholesterol. And all the tree nuts you will find in this book are high in unsaturated fat, which does not raise blood cholesterol and, when it replaces saturated fat, lowers blood cholesterol.

Another benefit of nuts in nutrition is that nuts are very low in saturated fats—fats that are an important contributor to high blood cholesterol, atherosclerosis, and coronary heart disease—and they do not contain cholesterol.

Nuts are good sources of plant fiber, plant sterols, and antioxidants. Both plant fiber and plant sterols can play a role in lowering cholesterol. Plant sterols are a much ignored element in human nutrition, which, even in low doses, have been shown to inhibit cholesterol absorption and have benefits in the prevention of coronary heart disease. Antioxidants may help prevent the oxidation of blood cholesterol, which is particularly harmful.

Not less important for people who are used to eating fatty foods, nuts can satisfy that desire when used as snacks to replace other fatty foods, such as cheese or butter. They can also add a burst of flavor to lower-fat, blander foods.

I have mentioned just a few of the many reasons why nuts should play an important, beneficial role in your diet. In this book, you will find facts that will place nuts in the proper light.

—John W. Farquhar, M.D.
Professor of Medicine and Director,
Stanford University Wellness Center

Preface

One day I set out in an earnest attempt to find the *good fats*. I tried to learn all I could about them: I set up clinical studies, I went to medical meetings, I read scientific publications, and I discussed diet and fats with the experts. That day I started on a long, tortuous journey to find out all I could about fat in the diet—how good or bad fats were for us and how much or how little of them we should consume. I discovered published papers in medical journals and medical books . . . but something wasn't quite right— something was missing.

There was something elusive about this whole picture. Scientists had made many discoveries about fats, and yet there were almost insurmountable gaps. The debate on how much or how little fat should be in the diet was far from over: all the researchers seemed to have a good point in their claims for lower or not-so-low fat consumption. Why then such a lack of agreement? What was missing in our knowledge, in our approach?

I felt I was caught up in a mystery, and the solution evaded me. Then the idea came to me that perhaps the current research on fats was good for expanding our basic scientific knowledge and as a valuable starting point, but it was not enough to give to the public sound recommendations on fats. It came to me that in everyday life, we eat whole, extremely complex foods containing hundreds of compounds, not isolated fats or proteins or carbohydrates.

In my search, nuts appeared to be a good example of a food that is extremely complex, very rich in a wide array of valuable compounds and, yes, certainly rich in good fats as well. Yet this great food was set aside by many people who thought of it as a high-fat food. This did not make sense at all, considering that in the 1980s researchers at Loma Linda University in California had found that most of those eating a handful of nuts a day had less heart disease than low or no nut eaters. Later, in a clinical study conducted at the Health Research and Studies Center—an organization, of which I am founder and director, dedicated to clinical nutritional studies—we fed lots of almonds to various groups of people with high blood cholesterol, and their cholesterol went down and *stayed down*. Since that time, many other studies have confirmed that nuts are a great and unique health food.

Nuts became for me a key example of the need to study whole foods in addition to single nutrients in isolation. It seemed to me that a book on nuts that was easy to read for everyone and that included their history, lore, and their role in a good diet and in good nutrition with as little medical jargon as possible was needed. Such a book could not only help find the proper place for nuts in our diets, but also help to bring about the idea that we should look at foods as a whole rather than making our choices based exclusively on single components. Basic research on individual components of foods is crucial, no doubt, but we must think in the context of whole foods, or generalization can confuse not only the general public but researchers as well.

As my search continued, I realized that nuts were not just an acceptable food, they were truly one of our superfoods, that not only can be, but should be part of our diet. I hope that you will find in this book concepts that go beyond nuts, concepts that give you the key to designing meals and snacks for ultimate health.

After reading this book, you'll never again judge the healthfulness of foods the same way. And you'll understand why foods should be judged in their totality, not just by focusing on a few isolated nutrients.

Introduction

Nuts are among the most fascinating foods we have, and this book will show that tree nuts are superfoods and among the healthiest foods. Tree nuts are ancient foods that have fed humanity through the ages, before the beginning of farming when people gathered food for survival. Later, as agriculture began to supply more and more of our staple foods, nuts continued to be an important part of the diet.

Then, in the second half of the twentieth century, something happened, and people, bombarded by messages that they should consume a diet low in fat, began to eat fewer nuts. For some people, nuts have become a food of doubtful healthful properties and an undesirable food rather than a treasure chest of good nutrition. Yes, nuts are superfoods, and this book will prove it. It's amazing that there is no popular book written exclusively about nuts that brings to the public the history, life, lore, and health benefits of tree nuts, with a major focus on the key role that nuts play in a good diet. At the beginning of a new millennium, nuts need to be re-established as a great healthful food.

Healthy Nuts will drive home the concept that there are *good* fats and that we should look at whole, unrefined foods, such as nuts, as the sum of a multitude of compounds, all with their special benefits. This book will show the reader the health benefits of nuts and how nuts should be a regular part of the diet. It will help to bring into focus the role of the good fats in the diet with quotes from leading researchers such as Drs. Walter Willett, (Harvard), Gary Fraser and Joan Sabaté, (Loma Linda University), Antonia Trichopoulou (University of Athens, Greece), David Jenkins (University of Toronto), and others.

Part One opens with the intriguing history of the early quest for food by primitive societies in Chapter 1. Later in this chapter, we follow nuts through the centuries, and we start our search for superfoods for the new millennium by discovering the power in a seed. But can a food fairly high in fat be a healthy food? In Chapter 2, we will untangle the fat maze and show that there are many good fats that not only can be but should be part of a healthy diet. You will learn that the ultimate way to consume these good fats is as part of whole plant foods such as nuts and seeds. Chapter 3 tells us about the benefits of other nutrients in nuts and how they interact with fats, reaching the conclusion that we should judge the healthfulness of a food by studying all of its components. Chapter 4 shows how nuts can be protective against chronic diseases with some stunning evidence from major population studies and controlled clinical research.

In Part Two, you will discover the origin of common tree nuts on every continent of the world not covered by ice. Each of the following chapters covers specific nuts: almonds, Brazil nuts, cashews, hazelnuts, macadamias, pecans, pine nuts, pistachios, and walnuts.

In Part Three, you will learn how to make nuts part of a healthy diet, with hints and suggestions on the uses of nuts.

I hope you enjoy reading this book as much as I enjoyed writing it, and that you walk away from it realizing just how important nuts are to a healthy, well-rounded diet.

PART ONE

Nuts in History
and Health

1

The Quest for Food

In the beginning, as the case is now, the first law of survival was that one must consume enough nutrients to stay alive, to feel strong, and to be able to be active. In that primitive society, men and women followed the laws of the wild. Wild plants supplied leaves, fruits, seeds, stems, and roots. The hunting of wild animals and the eating of their meats supplemented this plant-based diet, and as people moved farther and farther away from warm tropical and temperate climates, wild animals, by necessity, had to become an even more important part of life, as in cold climates, plants were not as easily accessible as they were in warm climates. As people moved closer to oceans, lakes, and streams, fish were often easy prey, were easy to prepare, and supplemented the nutrition that plants supplied.

Picture an early society in a tropical paradise where the people ate the pulp of sweet fruits or the leaves and stems of plants. Soon these people found out that these foods were not sufficient to give them enough energy and strength, and for their children to grow well. In those early days, before farming began to supply grains, beans, and other high-energy, nutrient-rich foods, one way to get other nutrients was to supplement the plant-food diet with the meat of land animals or fishes. It was soon discovered that meat supplied some substances—which we now call proteins—that were essential to the growth and maintenance of the body, and concentrated energy in what we now call fat. Obtaining these animal foods required hunting with primitive tools for an often elusive prey, or fishing. Weather conditions would often make hunting or fishing difficult, and no less troublesome was the fact that the flesh of these animals or fishes would quickly spoil. The meat of the killed animal had to be eaten soon, resulting often in a feast, followed by days without any meat at all.

Primitive humans needed an alternative to meats and fish. They needed foods that contained what we now call protein, fat, carbohydrates, vitamins, minerals, and other compounds that would round out the composition of leaves, fresh and dried fruits, roots, and stems. Just as important, they needed a protein-rich, high-energy food that would not quickly spoil as meats did.

In the days before farming began, while men were out hunting, with uncertain results, gathering green leaves, nuts, acorns, fruits, edible roots, flowers, and mushrooms was the task of the women. The wisdom of these ancient women not only saved these early societies from starvation, but also added to their diet that long list of protective compounds we find in foods from plants.

We can say with no fear of being found wrong that ancient women saved ancient men and that's why we are here today.

THE DISCOVERY OF NUTS

Soon the seeds of certain trees were discovered to contain substances that were essential to growth and maintenance. It was also quite likely that these seeds were found to have some extra health benefits, such as protection against some chronic diseases. The seeds of these trees are what we call *tree nuts* today.

Nuts could be consumed raw after breaking their shells with stones, and not less important to a primitive society, nuts came in a handy package—their hard shell—that protected them from spoilage, contamination, and insects for months. It seems as though nature wanted to protect one of its greatest nutrition-packed foods.

You may think of nuts as the first and most ancient of the protein- and energy-rich seeds. Others have been added as farming replaced the hunter-gatherer society. Together with nuts, these newer seeds are now the staples of humanity. These are the grains, legumes, beans, peas, peanuts, lentils, and oily seeds such as sesame and sunflower.

Ancient societies soon found out that nuts; the pulp of fruits; and the leaves, stems, and roots of plants not only made survival possible, but resulted in "superhealth."

A MODERN TRAGEDY

Somehow in recent decades, something tragic has happened. Strangely, the picture of nuts as superfoods in the minds of many people became blurred due to major misunderstandings about fats in the diet. This picture desperately needs proper refocusing.

The time has come for a voyage through time, space, and science to rediscover what tree nuts can do for us. Along our voyage, we'll encounter scientists and physicians who have been deeply involved in researching food and health. We'll discover the history, lore, and nutritional value of nuts, and why and how they not only can be but should be part of a healthy diet. And we'll learn what we need to do to make nuts a key part of our eating pattern.

During our voyage, let's never forget that only ancient foods, like nuts, have a long history of use, giving us a confidence we cannot have in newly created artificial products. Artificial products may be safe, they may even be good, but we may not know all we need to know about them for decades. Let's begin our voyage by learning the power that Nature has put in a seed and how nuts and seeds are superfoods.

POWER IN A SEED

"I have great faith in a seed. Convince me that you have a seed there, and I am prepared to expect wonders," wrote Thoreau in his last book, *Faith in a Seed*.

Consider this: From a seed, a new plant will grow, often a tree of majestic dimensions. To make this possible, it takes a package of many compounds that will, in the presence of water, allow the seed to sprout and live a life of its own for quite a while. What a powerful package a little seed must be to make possible the birth of a tree. Look at the ground in a forest of pine trees: the pine cones filled with pine nuts fall, and the cones release the pine nuts. The cones slowly decompose, some pine nuts feed squirrels and other wild animals. The oils in the nuts give these animals glossy fur and all the nutrients combined give them bodybuilding substances and the energy for their active lives. Squirrels bury a few pine nuts to eat later, but some of these sprout, and gigantic pine trees grow from them. Is there any doubt that there is tremendous hidden power in a seed?

Of the seeds that are a common part of the human diet, tree nuts and whole grains are tremendous storehouses of balanced energy, good fats, proteins, vitamins, minerals, and a large number of other compounds that scientists have recently found to be so protective against disease, called *phytochemicals* (*phyto*, Greek for plant). These compounds are superprotective—scientists like to call them bioactive, that is, biologically active—against a variety of damages to our bodies. Thousands of these phytochemicals are in natural foods from plants. Until a few years ago, we thought that these compounds were good only for coloring or flavoring.

BEYOND FOODS: DEFINING NATURAL SUPERFOODS

Let's see how a food can be classified as a superfood. While there are many good foods available to us, superfoods are foods that are super-rich in a variety of precious and valuable components. After extensive discussions with various researchers, I have established four basic requirements that a food must meet in order to be considered a superfood:

1. They must have a long history of use.

2. They must be rich in a variety of biologically healthy compounds.

3. They must not have a significant amount of any compounds that should not be part of the diet.

4. They must be palatable and easy to prepare.

   Think of a superfood as a food rich in good proteins, good fats, carbohydrates, fiber, vitamins, precious minerals, and phytochemicals.

Tree Nuts as Superfoods

Has nature created such foods? Yes, such superfoods do exist, and a few foods from plants qualify for this prestigious award of "superfood." Some of them need some preparation, like wheat needs to be baked into a precious loaf of whole-grain bread; others are ready to eat, not needing cooking, with their own shell to protect them and keep them fresh for long-time storage. There is no doubt that one such superfood is the *tree nut* in its many varieties and forms.

Humans and animals learned quickly to eat nuts and to store them. They learned to combine them with other seeds, leaves, stems, roots, and fruits in what was probably the most ancient diet of the human race in temperate and tropical climates. Watch the squirrel in your garden, watch how she climbs your nut tree and picks that ripe nut, takes it along to her home and stores it carefully.

Tree nuts today sit together with other superhealthy foods, many of which entered the history of humanity as farming began to replace the gathering of wild plant products. Nature in her wisdom has put nuts in all regions of the world so that, in the days before modern transportation, all people could use them as one of their basic foods.

Now that we have placed tree nuts on such a high pedestal, let's not forget that in planning our diets, even such superfoods as nuts and other seeds need to be combined with foods derived from other parts of the plant, such as leaves, fruits, roots, and flowers, to give us a healthy diet. This is a key concept for a healthy diet.

One great advantage for our fast-moving modern society is that nuts are a superfood, ready to eat as they come from the tree. Dr. Joan Sabaté of Loma Linda University's Department of Nutrition reminds us of this great advantage of nuts:

> *Nuts are a food that nature has created in a way that they are ready to be consumed without cooking. Eating nuts could be*

*an easy way to get a well-rounded diet, without spending
hours and hours in the kitchen in food preparation.*

*But nuts are a group of foods that somehow have been put
aside or forgotten by the general public for several reasons.
Nuts are an essential constituent of most traditional diets,
from the Middle Eastern to the European to the Indian diet,
and I think these lapses in the twentieth century of not using
nuts as they were used in the past probably will only be lapses
in the sense that more nuts will be used as the knowledge about
their benefits becomes known. Nuts are an easy and conven-
ient source of many nutrients that we need in the diet.*

The Nutritional Power of a Tree Nut

In this book, you'll learn why tree nuts are such a valuable food.
But before we learn all about tree nuts, we need to dispel many of
the misunderstandings about fat in the diet, as tree nuts do supply
some very good fats, fats that carry many healthful compounds.

2

Untangling the Fat Maze

I n unrefined foods, components such as fats, proteins, carbohydrates, fiber, vitamins, minerals, and phytochemicals do not
live lives of their own in isolation. While studies of isolated
compounds are essential to our better understanding of the
healthy or unhealthy properties of a food, the final benefit or harm
of a food comes from the sum of all the components of that food.
We need to consider each natural food as a marvelous complex of
a myriad of compounds. Nutrients do not live in an isolated cabin,
separated from the rest of the world by heavy winter snowstorms.
And nutrients interact with nutrients in other foods to create a
beautiful, harmonious and life-giving picture. Furthermore, we
need to judge any food in the context of the total diet. If you
remember these key concepts as you choose your foods, you'll
have made a major step toward better health.

Some important, healthful foods, like nuts, many seeds, avocados, and olives, are often relegated to the wrong place in our diets
because of their fat content. Let's look at fats first in this chapter
and, later, in Chapter 3, at how other components of a food make
the difference in the final health outcome.

FATS: EVIL OR BLESSING?

For years, consumers have labored under the assumption that

"fat" is the most evil three-letter word in their everyday diet. "The lower the fat, the better the diet" has become the mantra, and keeping fats out of the diet is supposedly the greatest thing people can do for their health. Food manufacturers and packaged-goods companies have made billions of dollars selling their products on the basis of "low-fat," "reduced-fat," or "nonfat" advertising.

Like a dark cloud hovering over our dinner table, the concept that fat is intrinsically bad has cast a shadow over our joy of eating for many years. There are two basic flaws in this approach to fats. The first is that though we have been led to believe that all fats are bad, there are many diverse kinds of fats in foods, some not only acceptable but even good. The second flaw is that we have been flooded with reports that have led to the strange concept that there is either a *low-fat* or a *high-fat* diet. Have you ever thought it strange that there is nothing between *low* and *high*? If you thought of this in terms of money, it would be as if the only options were for you to be either poor or a millionaire.

Go to a market and look at a food label, read a magazine, or listen to an ad on TV, and it will appear to you that the single message is to reduce your fat intake. It's like a bad dream: There is a mania, an obsession, to lower fat in one's diet. It has become almost a sin to put some olive oil on a salad, to enjoy some walnuts or almonds, or to eat an avocado. Is this right? Is Nature an evil, vicious, wicked entity that has put fat in so many of our great natural seeds and fruits and thus laid the foundation for many killer diseases? Saying "fat is bad" is like saying that some plants are poisonous (very true), so all plant foods are poisonous (fortunately false, or no animal or human being would be alive today).

See the inset on page 13, "Test Your Fat IQ." Take this quiz now before reading more of this chapter to see just how much you know about fats. Then take the quiz again after reading this chapter.

CHANGING THE WAY WE LOOK AT FATS

As you read this book, you'll realize that plant fats are a key component of the diet. Here are some surprising answers to many crucial issues on diet, fats, disease prevention, and body weight:

Test Your Fat I.Q.

Everyone seems to oversimplify the effects of fats. But it's really not all that simple. Take this test to see just how much you know about fats. Mark each question with an answer of either True (T) or False (F).

1. *One should stay away from all fats as much as possible.*

2. *All saturated fats raise blood cholesterol.*

3. *Polyunsaturated fats are essential to health.*

4. *Monounsaturated fats are very safe for us, no matter what type.*

5. *Only fats and cholesterol in food affect the level of our blood cholesterol.*

6. *Antioxidants like vitamin E play an important role in the way fat affects our health.*

7. *For a healthy person, too little fat can be just as bad as too much.*

8. *Peasants in some Mediterranean countries consume a reasonable amount of olive oil and nuts and have some of the lowest rates of heart disease in the world.*

9. *Too little fat can lower our good blood cholesterol.*

10. *Margarines high in trans-fatty acids are much safer than butter.*

Answers:
1. F; 2. F; 3. T; 4. F; 5. F; 6. T; 7. T; 8. T; 9. T; 10. F

- There are *good* fats that should definitely be a part of our diets, just as there are fats we should keep low in our diet.

- There are no natural bad fats, a shocking fact to many.

- The good fats can be a part of a good disease-and-overweight-prevention program.

- The good fats can bring joy to our meals.

- We do not have to try to eat as little fat as possible.

- Many non-fat components of foods alter the way fats affect our health.

NUTRITION LABELS ON FOODS

Nutrition labels serve a very useful purpose: They let us know what we are eating. But food labels seem to have made everybody think of fat as "bad," or at least unnecessary, and the terms "reduced-fat" and "low-fat" in prepared foods are taken to indicate the best possible thing that could happen to a food. These statements on labels have led too many people to think that fat is intrinsically bad, and the lower its level in your diet, the better off you are. While some of these reduced-fat foods, such as low-fat milk, yogurt, and cheeses, can be very useful in planning your diet, what has happened is that people are using these labels as a license to eat as much of these foods as possible. Not only that, but these labels make you think that the lower the fat, the healthier the food. This misconception has caused many natural foods, like nuts and many other seeds, avocados, and olives—that not only have been part of the human diet for millennia, but often have been considered sacred—to be considered bad for us.

ARE LOW-FAT FOODS HELPING?

Notwithstanding all the food labels and the processed reduced-fat foods on the supermarket shelves, there are more overweight people than ever in many Western countries, including the United States. It is not because there aren't some great low-fat or fat-free foods in nature, like many fresh and dried fruits, vegetables, whole grains, lentils, and beans, but because we have created so many processed foods that people believe can be consumed in unlimited quantities.

The natural, high-fat plant foods, such as many nuts, fruits like avocados and olives, and seeds like sesame, which have good fats balanced by a large number of valuable compounds, are dumped together in a large box with all kinds of high-fat foods that should be consumed in limited quantities or left out of the diet altogether.

"Until quite recently that three-letter word [fat] had a decidedly positive connotation," wrote Jane Brody in the 1996 Christmas issue of *The New York Times*. "[But] in the last few years the country has gone hog wild over low-fat, non-fat and fat-free foods. Supermarket shelves groan with cakes, cookies, chips, dips, cheese, sausage and that quintessential no-no, ice cream, minus most or all of the fat. People think that by avoiding fat, they will automatically shed pounds. But many who once ate sparingly of such foods now indulge freely in their low-fat or non-fat versions, sometimes downing servings two or three times as large as those they would eat of the full-fat food. As a result, many Americans desperate to shrink their widening girth are getting fatter still on fat-free foods and little or no exercise. The recent introduction of snack foods prepared with an indigestible fat, Olestra, is likely to feed the desire to 'have one's cake and eat it too' even further without doing a single thing to improve Americans' dietary habits."

Another writer, Laura Shapiro, in a *Newsweek* cover story in December 1994, asked if America's fat-free food obsession had gone too far. We now know that, in fact, we have gone too far. You do not have to be a statistician to look at the facts and see that as low-fat foods become more and more available, the percentage of overweight people goes up instead of down. Some say that fat-free foods become a license for overeating and are consumed too freely. But this is only part of the truth: The human body needs some fat and craves it. A few nuts can make you feel satisfied quickly, and you actually eat less in the long run.

AN OVERWEIGHT EPIDEMIC EVEN WITH LOW-FAT FOODS

The number of overweight men and women in the United States, which had hardly changed at all from 1960 to the late 1970s (although it was too high even in those years) has increased dramatically from the late 1970s to early 1990s, from about 24 percent in 1970 to 34 percent in the early 1990s. In the 1970s, almost one-quarter of the United States population was overweight, and in the early 1990s, about one-third was overweight. This means that the number of overweight men and women has increased by over 30 percent.

In the same period, the number of low-fat or reduced-fat foods increased tremendously in the United States. As more low-fat foods are available to the public, the trend should lead to fewer overweight people, right? Well, this has not been the case. And as more people go on weight-loss diets, these diets often fail. A short-lived success is followed by a relapse and greater weight gain by the poor dieter. Major popular magazines, from *Newsweek* to *Time* to *Life*, have had cover stories in recent years about the overweight American population.

Is this overweight epidemic just an American phenomenon? Drs. Barry Popkin and Colleen Doak of the University of North Carolina have studied trends in obesity and overweight in many countries and have written that obesity is a worldwide phenomenon, not just a disease of developed countries. And they add that the percentage of the population that is overweight in many lower-income and developing countries is rapidly increasing. But the United States retains the dubious distinction of being one of the most overweight countries.

This is tragic. Excess weight is known to be more than just an issue of appearance, it can be outright dangerous. Obesity is indeed a disease. We now know that overweight men and women are not just unfit; they are at a much greater risk for heart disease, diabetes, high blood pressure, and even cancer. More and more research is confirming these close links between chronic diseases and overweight. Yet, some people consider overweight to be just an aesthetic problem!

Discussing low-fat diets, JoAnn Harmer, a Stanford University dietitian, reminded us that, "Nonfat foods clear out of your stomach more quickly and you're hungry faster. So you may eat more." It's well known that carbohydrates leave the stomach very rapidly when little or no fat is present. When refined carbohydrates, such as pasta and white bread, are consumed without fiber, the feeling of satiety is even less. No doubt, most Americans eat a low-fiber diet despite all the talk about the benefits of fiber. The feeling of satiety comes from fat in the diet, as well as from fiber. In cholesterol-lowering studies conducted at our Center in the San Francisco Bay area (see page 47), when we fed about three ounces of almonds a day to a group of subjects for a few weeks, many of the subjects were afraid that they might gain weight. No one gained weight, and many subjects felt so well satisfied that they actually ate fewer calories than they had eaten on their previous low-fat diets.

TYPES OF FATS

Is it possible that Nature has not created any bad fats? Could it be that perhaps in our sincere desire to improve people's diets, we have created a false concept that there are bad fats in an absolute sense? Take the much-maligned saturated fats—how unwise Nature would have been if these fats were bad for us in an absolute sense, as there is practically no natural food from either plants or animals that is totally free from saturated fats, often referred to as "bad fats." With this premise in mind, let's learn more about the different types of fat.

Saturated Fats

Fat molecules are chains of various lengths with many atoms linked in many ways. The way the atoms are linked to each other makes a great deal of difference in their effects on our bodies. When all of the bonds in the fat are very stable, such that you cannot insert much else in the bond—it's full already—and hard to break, the fat is called saturated. Saturated fats are usually a major constituent of the fat found in animal products, with the exception of fish, which is low in saturated fat. Coconut is one the few plant foods high in saturated fat. Keep your intake of saturated fats low. You'll get enough no matter what you eat. There is some saturated fat in all the fats we consume, whether it comes from animals or plants. The difference is in the amount of saturated fats, compared to the unsaturated fats.

Certain types of saturated fats, when taken in sufficient

amounts, raise blood cholesterol, a fact made worse when the saturated fat comes from animal products such as meats, as these foods also contain cholesterol. An exception to this rule is a saturated fat called *stearic acid*, the main fat in cocoa beans. This fat does not raise blood cholesterol, which is good news for chocolate lovers. Keep the amount of meats and poultry low in your diet, and use low-fat milk products. Limit your intake of higher-fat milk products, such as regular cheeses, to occasional use and as flavorings, for example, using Parmesan cheese on pasta.

Long chains of saturated fat, sometimes with eighteen or twenty bonds, can change in a major way if we insert just one or two or three unsaturated bonds along the way. Chemists call these unsaturated bonds in a fat molecule *double bonds*. Inserting one double bond makes the fat monounsaturated (*mono* means one), inserting more than one double bond makes it polyunsaturated (*poly* means many). In this book, I'll often refer to the monounsaturated fats as the *monos* and the polyunsaturated fats as the *polys*.

Natural Monounsaturated Fats

Natural monounsaturated fats are the basic fats of the healthy Mediterranean diets of Southern Italy, Greece, the Middle East, and North Africa. When monounsaturated fats replace saturated fats in the diet, they lower blood cholesterol, and they do not favor harmful oxidation (damage by hyperactive oxygen) in the arteries of the heart and other arteries, which makes the bad cholesterol worse. The mono fats are not very sensitive to oxygen damage. Little wonder that these should be the predominant fats in the diet. Most of the nuts I'll describe later contain this type of fat as their major fat.

Synthetic Hydrogenated, Trans-Monounsaturated Fats

Hydrogenated fats are mono fats, which are supposed to be good fats. The trouble is that during processing, their molecule becomes twisted. Margarines based on this type of fat were at one point in time considered a great thing for your heart and much healthier than butter. People who wanted to avoid animal fat thought this was great.

Hydrogenated fats are made from vegetable oils that are made artificially solid by adding hydrogen to the molecule under special chemical conditions. As a result, the fat becomes solid, and the molecule becomes twisted. Nobody thought much about this until 1990, when Drs. M. Katan and R. Mensink in the Netherlands published an article in a medical journal that made headlines. They proved that these fats were actually worse for your heart than natural saturated fats.

Dr. Walter Willett, a professor and chair of the department of nutrition at Harvard University's School of Public Health, is one of the key researchers in some of the largest studies on diet and health, including the often quoted Nurses Study. He feels strongly about this kind of fat:

> *The key players in the area of fats that have been neglected—in fact covered up—are trans fatty acids—which are produced by the partial hydrogenation of liquid vegetable fats, which turns them into margarine. But now, probably even more importantly, they're the types of fat used for the deep-frying of fast foods and also the types of fat that are used very widely in commercial baked products. On food labels, they are often listed as "partially hydrogenated fats." On an ounce-per-ounce basis, trans fatty acids have about twice the bad effect on blood lipids as do saturated fats, because they both raise the LDL or bad cholesterol and also reduce the HDL or good cholesterol. Moreover, the epidemiological studies—studies of large population groups where we follow the diet and the health of the people for long periods—really suggest that trans fats are even worse than you would anticipate, by their very bad effects on blood lipids. The relationship with coronary heart disease risk actually seems to be greater than you would predict just by the metabolic studies.*
>
> *We do know that there are additional bad effects with trans fats: they do raise blood triglyceride [a type of fat found in the blood] levels. No other fat does that, and they also raise a lipoprotein called "little a," [lp(a)] which has been recently*

added to the list of blood factors that have a [causative] relationship with heart disease. Again, no other type of fat does that. So we already know that there are some extra bad things that trans fatty acids do. They are hidden in our food supply. A lot of people oftentimes think they're making a healthy choice, and they're being badly misled because [trans fatty acids] are not even on the food label.

Polyunsaturated Fats

In polyunsaturated fats, the molecule contains more unsaturated bonds. There are many kinds of poly fats with two or more of these bonds. Poly fats are essential to health as they are the raw material for the synthesis of key compounds in the body, such as the powerful prostaglandins that control many body functions. Poly fats lower blood cholesterol. But they are very active in a chemical sense, and because of this, they are very easily oxidized. These fats always need to be taken together with compounds that prevent oxidation, such as vitamin E and many other antioxidants (compounds that combat oxidation's effects). This means that we can feel freer to use poly fats when they are part of whole foods, such as walnuts, one of the few common tree nuts high in polyunsaturated fats, or of oils high in antioxidants. They are even safer if we eat them with plenty of antioxidant-rich vegetables and fruits such as carrots, yellow squashes, and dark green leaves. If you use polyunsaturated oils, be sure they are unrefined, with their natural antioxidants present!

A special type of polyunsaturated fat comes from fish and some plants. They are referred to as omega-3 fats. Among tree nuts, walnuts are a good source. Omega-3 fats have become so popular that concentrates are now available as supplements. Populations consuming these fats have lower rates of heart disease, a fact probably related to their power to prevent abnormal blood coagulation that leads to the formation of deadly blood clots in blood vessels.

Watch out for hidden fats. Baked products, including pastries and breads; cereals; frozen dinners; and canned foods can be a source of hidden fats. Solid fats—that is, saturated or hydrogenated fats—are a favorite of pastry chefs and of the food industry. They are, it is said, *functional fats,* meaning they help improve the way the food feels in the mouth and the way it behaves during cooking and other processing.

HEALTHY ANCIENT DIETS

We forget that the regular diets in many regions of the world, where some of the major Western chronic killer diseases—heart disease and cancer—are very low, are not low in fat. Typical are the diets of some Asian countries; Crete, a Greek island; Southern Italy; the Middle East; and many Mediterranean countries. In all these regions, plant foods high in unsaturated fats are a key part of the diet.

The fact that foods containing reasonable amounts of good fats are not only acceptable but healthy is seen in the high esteem in which many such foods were held through the ages. To confirm that a diet moderate in fat can be healthy, let's look at some Mediterranean diets, where olive oil is used as a basic staple. Take the olive: an ancient food, highly regarded in these Mediterranean countries for millennia. Large groves of olive trees in the Middle East already existed before Christ, and in the Bible, olive groves are often mentioned: "For the Lord your God is bringing you into a good land—a land with streams and pools of water, with springs flowing in the valleys and hills; a land with wheat and barley, vines and fig trees, pomegranates, *olive* oil and honey." (Deuteronomy 8:7)

Olives are similar to many nuts in the type of fat they contain, and they are part of one of the healthiest diets in the world, the Greek diet. The consumption of olives with their good fats in the Greek population, which has a low occurrence of cancer and heart disease, gives additional support to the use of foods such as nuts. Here is Dr. Antonia Trichopoulou, from the University of Athens in Greece, on olives.

In Greece we eat a lot of olives. Sometimes we add them to salad; sometimes we eat them as a snack with bread. And we use them to make an olive bread, as they do in Southern Italy, another region with low rates of heart disease. We make an olive paste that we put on bread. So mainly we eat them with bread in various ways.

We found out that Greek postmenopausal women who consume olive oil more than once per day have lower risk for breast cancer. Olive oil is similar to the oils found in many nuts. The results of this important study have been published in a major British medical journal, Lancet.

There is an ancient village on the side of a hill in Umbria in central Italy. The sweeping view of grapevines, olive groves, nut trees, and fields of fruits and vegetables down in the valley below are reminiscent of the paintings of fourteenth-century Italian Renaissance masters.

The people of this town remind us that natural fats from plant foods can be part of a healthy diet. They eat a frugal diet that includes nuts, fruits, vegetables, beans, and grains and use olive oil pressed in an old-fashioned local press. I met a man who was about eighty-five years old, but he looked fifty-five or sixty. His skin was smooth, his mind bright, and he had never seen a physician in his life. "Most people here," he says, "live to be ninety or even 100 years old." Then he took me to an ancient olive press. "The people of the town gather their own olives from the trees on the hills around here. They bring the olives in and watch the pressing. Usually they mix some olive leaves with the olives as well—this is an ancient custom. Then, they store this oil carefully and drink some in the morning—a few tablespoons in a glass—while they eat some cereal and bread. They use olive oil throughout the day, day after day. I don't know if it's true, but I think this oil is one of the things that keeps us healthy." As I looked around, I saw that no one was overweight! There is no hard scientific evidence about the life history of the people of this town, but I feel there is a great deal of truth in this story.

Why these stories about olive oil in a book about nuts? Because it reinforces the concept that natural fats from fruits and seeds can be part of a healthy diet and reminds us that many ancient, healthy diets are not very low in fat.

FEWER STROKES WITH HIGHER FAT INTAKE?

A study of 832 initially healthy middle-aged men, conducted by Dr. Matthew W. Gillman of the Harvard Medical School and published in the *Journal of the American Medical Association* in December 1997, showed that healthy men who participated in the long-term Framingham Heart Study, in Framingham, Massachusetts, and ate a higher-fat diet in the 1960s were less likely to suffer a stroke caused by a blood clot that got stuck in a brain blood vessel. Vice versa, those in the study who consumed the lowest amount of fat had the highest stroke risk. Further study is needed to find the reason for this.

While both saturated fats and monounsaturated fats showed the same relationship to this lower occurrence of strokes, an excess (remember, *excess* only) of some types of saturated fats could lead to heart disease. So the wise choice is foods high in mono- or poly-fats, such as nuts. Again this study shows the wisdom of Mediterranean-type diets, which are moderate but not low in fat and high in fruits and vegetables, grains, and nuts.

HOW MUCH FAT SHOULD THERE BE IN OUR DIETS?

When you hear or read about the amount of fat in a food or in the diet, it is usually given in the percentage of calories from fat compared with calories from proteins and carbohydrates. Calories from fat are usually 30 to 40 percent in typical diets. Should it be less or not? Is 30 percent better than 40 percent, or is much lower better? I have asked some experts, like Dr. Gary Fraser from Loma Linda University, Dr. Walter Willett from Harvard and Dr. John Farquhar from Stanford.

Dr. Gary Fraser of Loma Linda University conducted a study on 34,000 people of diet and health, called the Adventist Health Study. Here is what Dr. Fraser has to say:

> As a group, the fat consumption of the people in our study was not particularly low; just a little lower than the general population, but only by probably 2 or 3 percent. We're not talking here about a low-fat-consuming population. I think the differ-

ence is the kinds of fat. The nut consumers tended to eat more of the mono- and polyunsaturated fats, which, of course, are the main type of fat of nuts. The amount of fat they consumed was still the typical amount of fat, about 30 to 35 percent, or maybe even more than that. We don't necessarily need to eat a very low-fat diet to have lower risk of heart disease. From our study, it appears that the type of fat is much more important than the quantity of fat.

How much fat should we eat? Dr. Walter Willett, Chair of the Department of Nutrition of Harvard University, thinks that clinical studies are unequivocally clear that 30 percent is less good than 40 percent, if that 40 percent is from good and nonhydrogenated vegetable fats. As you read Dr. Willett's suggestions below for the amount of fat that should make up your diet, focus on a key point, a point I am making over and over again: fats do not live in isolation. You just can't say X-amount of fat is good or is too much or is too little: It all depends on the rest of the diet. When a health professional tells you in absolute terms that so much of something is good or bad without taking into account the rest of your diet and your physical activity, her or his view is too limited to be credible. Here is what Dr. Willet says:

> *I think it's not fully clear what the optimal level of fat is in the diet, and I think that should suggest to us that [the amount of fat is] probably not the most important thing, first of all, that there's probably a very wide range of fat intakes that are compatible with very healthy diets. So it's more [important that] if you're eating fat, eat healthy fat; if you're eating carbohydrate, eat a healthy carbohydrate, eating plenty of fruits and vegetables to go along with it. However, having said that, it [healthy levels of intake] also depends on the population. If the population is very lean, very active, or if the individual is very lean and very active, they can tolerate a higher-carbohydrate, lower-fat diet. But the reality is that most of us in contemporary United States [and other] Western populations, even now in many parts of developing countries where there's a lot of urbanization—are not physically active most of the time.*

24

We're either [sitting] in school, [or] we sit at work, so even if we run three to four miles a day, we're still physically inactive most of the time, and for most of us that means that we're not going to be able to tolerate high-carbohydrate loads as well as we could if we were very lean and active, working in the fields all day long. So I look at the metabolic data and it's very clear to me that the higher-fat diet gives better results. There's absolutely no question about the metabolic results as long as that fat is a good fat, so that tempts me more to go with a higher fat Mediterranean-type pattern for most people. I think the metabolic data very strongly brings you in that direction — perhaps around 40 percent of calories from fat.

According to Dr. John Farquhar, Professor of Medicine at Stanford University:

For most people, fat should not go below 25 percent of calories from fat, perhaps 30 or 35 percent is better if we are talking plant-based diets. What I mean is, the percent of calories from fat depends on the source of fat. If we are talking fats from animal sources, this amount of fat would be way too much. I think that's where the problem began, I mean the recommendations for very-low-fat diets. They assumed that much of the fat came from animal sources. And much of this fat should come from whole foods, like the original seed or nut rather than the oil that was derived from the food.

It is clear that the amount of fat in the diet is closely linked to the type of fat being taken in, to the rest of the diet, and to whether the fat is part of a whole food like nuts or seeds. On a plant-based diet and with a reasonable amount of physical activity, from 25 to 40 percent of energy from fats may be ideal for a healthy person. Many researchers focus on 30 to 35 percent. In the real world, anything between 25 and 40 percent appears healthy. What's important is that a large portion of this fat must come from whole foods like nuts and other seeds or fruits. Nuts can help design a healthy plant-based diet, as they satisfy hunger and contain enough proteins, fiber, and protective compounds. Nuts fit well in diets with a wide range of fat content, be it a 25-, 30-, or 40-percent fat diet.

To feel satisfied, we need some fat in our meals. When fat consumption is too low, the digestive system does not feel satisfied and sends signals to the brain asking for more food. Likewise, the digestive system quickly feels satisfied with a reasonable fat intake and tells the brain that no more food is needed.

Consumers want the taste of fat, and the food industry has developed some artificial compounds that taste like fat and often have the same characteristic when used in cooking. But these compounds are not digested nor do they have very low caloric content. Olestra is such a compound and gives chips and other snack foods that satisfying feeling. Olestra has been the center of much controversy, as it dissolves some critical oil-soluble compounds like vitamin A, and it is not absorbed, so as it goes through the digestive system it carries these precious compounds with it and eventually out of the body.

Suffering day after day on a fat-deprived diet is not going to work for too long. These diets have a proper place in special clinical cases, when disease has progressed to a point that a drastic diet may be needed, perhaps under professional supervision. But for the rest of us, the joy of eating is a crucial part of life. A student of mine at a San Francisco Bay Area college, a husky 24-year-old football player planning to go to graduate school, had high cholesterol. He decided to stop eating all foods containing more than a minimal amount of fat. At the end of the course, during a session when all students were asked to talk about personal experiences in nutrition, he told how, after a few weeks on this extreme diet, he went out to a fast-food restaurant and ate all the high-fat foods he could possibly find . . . some of them high in saturated animal fat. His body had rebelled against his eating too little fat!

After all that's been said about fats, we must remember that fats can be overeaten just like the best of carbohydrates, proteins, vitamins, and minerals and other key factors in our diet. We must balance these higher-fat foods with other superfoods from plants to arrive at the ultimate diet. And a key message to always remember: the amount of fat in the diet does not mean much unless you consider it in the context of the other foods you eat. We'll learn more about this in the next chapter.

FAT INTAKE AND PHYSICAL ACTIVITY

Diet is only a part of good health—as crucial as it may be. The human body must be physically active. Total health and disease prevention are not based on diet alone. Before we go any further, we need to realize that there are no good fats that can be "good" without some regular physical activity. This point is crucial for anyone, no matter how much or how little fat you eat. The human body was meant to be physically active, and this point should never be forgotten. People who exercise feel better and look better, and this should be an additional stimulus to being physically active.

In past centuries, wealthy people did not have to be physically active. Many of us are still not willing to accept the need for regular physical activity, a major reason for the growing problem of obesity in many Western countries. Consider how wise nature is: physical activity not only results in a healthier heart and better overall health, but it makes us look fit and relaxes and regenerates the mind. No food works well without physical activity.

Let's now look at how other compounds together with fats make a food more or less desirable for ultimate health and fitness.

3

What's in a Nutshell?

The edible part of a tree nut is the delicate, flavorful seed that we find inside the nut's hard shell. Often the hard shell with the seed inside is surrounded by a soft pulp—the husk. The thickness of the soft outer cover varies. Some fruits that are related to nuts, like the peach and the apricot, have an outer layer so thick that it is the part we usually eat—the fleshy fruit; but crack the stone of a peach, and the edible seed inside looks like an almond. Other nuts have no soft outer layer, like acorns—the nut of the oak tree—or hazelnuts. Pine nuts are found in the pine cone. But all tree nuts have in common a precious seed inside a hard protective shell.

Each nut is a storehouse of goodness. Don't be tempted to say that one is better than another. Differences in the amount of fats, protein, carbohydrates and fiber make each nut valuable for specific uses. In this chapter, we'll look at all common tree nuts together, comparing their basic nutrients: protein, fats, carbohydrates and fiber, phytochemicals, vitamins, and minerals.

THE NUTRIENTS IN NUTS

In the early days of modern nutrition, at the beginning of the twentieth century, when the first vitamin had just been discovered—vitamin B—Sir Robert McCarrison, a prestigious British physician, in his 1921 book, *Studies in Deficiency Disease*, wrote "The high value of groundnuts, almonds, walnuts, filberts [hazelnuts], Brazil nuts, chestnuts, hickory and pine nuts is due as much to the nutritive value of their protein as to their content of vitamin B."

Today, as we look inside the edible part of a nut, we find a large number of valuable compounds, far beyond the ones McCarrison wrote about in 1921. And with more research on the composition of nuts, we can expect more exciting data to become available in the next few years.

Let's first look at the major nutrients: fats, proteins, carbohydrates, and fiber. Then we will explore the major vitamins, minerals, and phytochemicals present in nuts. The values that are given represent the amount present after the water in the nuts has been removed. Water, what chemists call *moisture*, is usually very low in nuts—about 3 to 6 percent.

It does not take much effort to see that there are many similarities, and yet some major differences, among nuts. Keep in mind that data on food composition, as found in food tables and in this book, are averages that vary somewhat with soil, climate, and variety. Figures for nutrients are given in either percentages, that is the amount of grams of the given nutrient in a hundred grams—slightly more than three ounces—of the given nut, or the amount contained in an ounce—about 28 grams—of nuts. An ounce is a useful amount, as it's about a handful for most nuts.

As you read the values for various nutrients in nuts or any other food, you may think that you have seen somewhat different values somewhere else, perhaps on a food label or in another book. Tables of food composition are derived from averaging chemical analyses on many samples of a food. All values that follow should be considered typical, but subject to minor variations from region to region, soil to soil, and even year to year.

PLANT PROTEINS

Plant proteins are made up of different percentages of their building blocks—the amino acids—than are animal proteins. This could be one reason why people on plant-based diets usually have lower cholesterol. In a study we conducted at the Health Research and Studies Center (an organization I founded and direct, committed to clinical nutritional studies), we gave all subjects the same type and amount of fat, but some subjects were given plant protein—in this case a nut protein—and others were given animal protein. The nut diet lowered cholesterol much more effectively than the animal protein diet. This had been shown long ago, in the late 1970s, by Dr. David Kritchevsky of the Wistar Institute in Philadelphia. He compared casein, a milk protein, to a plant protein and found that, in laboratory animals, the plant protein resulted in lower cholesterol levels. The effect may be due to the presence of the little-talked-about amino acid *arginine*. This amino acid is much higher in nuts and plants than in common animal protein foods.

Some researchers speculate that the relative amount of arginine to another amino acid—lysine—is one reason for the beneficial effect of plant proteins on blood cholesterol. In 1982, Dr. Kritchevsky studied various proteins with different ratios of arginine to lysine and found a progressive increase in narrowing of the aorta—the large artery that carries blood from the heart to various other arteries that bring blood to various parts of the body—as the amount of arginine increased for a given level of lysine.

But arginine does more for us: it makes possible the synthesis of a compound, *nitric oxide*, which widens blood vessels and relaxes them. Nitric oxide is a very simple compound made up of nitrogen and oxygen, and it relaxes the blood vessel walls. Because of this property, it has been called *endothelium-derived relaxing factor*. The endothelium is the name for the layer of cells that line arteries. Nitric oxide's role in disease prevention and treatment is so important that the 1998 Nobel Prize for Medicine was awarded to the researchers that have shown its role in disease prevention.

This relaxation of blood vessels is often impaired in people with high cholesterol, even before cholesterol deposits begin to narrow the arteries. This does not happen to people with normal cholesterol. Dr. Peter Clarkson and his colleagues in London confirmed this relaxing effect of arginine in blood vessels by feeding an arginine supplement to volunteers. These researchers believe that arginine may have a favorable impact on preventing deposits of cholesterol in the arteries. The high-cholesterol group in this study showed a relaxation effect on the arteries of the arm, while the individuals with normal cholesterol did not.

There is another possible benefit of proteins with a high level of arginine: they may protect against formation of abnormal blood clots inside the blood vessels—thrombi, in medical jargon—clots that may get caught in an artery clogged by cholesterol deposits and cause a heart attack or a stroke. This possible role of arginine in heart disease prevention reminds us of the risk of focusing only on so-called "essential" nutrients, as arginine is one of the nonessential amino acids. This fact about arginine is another reason to increase the consumption of plant proteins and to avoid focusing only on types of fat in the diet when we think about heart disease.

It is possible that nitric oxide may have a connection with healthy sexual function in males. Many factors are involved, but while more studies are needed, certainly a diet with foods high in arginine, and the nitric oxide that arginine makes possible, could be part of maintaining normal sexual function. As I have said, more research is needed to determine the role of high-arginine foods in sexual function.

Protein in tree nuts ranges from about 5.7 grams in an ounce (20 percent) in almonds and pistachios to about 2.3 grams in an ounce (8 percent) in macadamia nuts and pecans.

If we compare the amount of arginine in nuts to some animal products for the same amount of total protein, we find that beef protein contains between 300 and 450 milligrams of arginine, and milk protein contains about 250 milligrams, while nuts range from 600 to 900 milligrams. That's two-and-a-half to three-and-a-half times as much as milk proteins. Arginine is another reason we should get some of our protein from nuts.

FATS

Despite fat's bad reputation, it is important to obtain some fats in your diet, particularly the "good" fats present in nuts. (See Chapter 2 to learn more about the benefits of some fats in your diet.) Fat content varies from about 19 to 20 grams per ounce (about 70 percent) in macadamia nuts to about 13 to 14 grams per ounce (46 to 50 percent) in cashew nuts and pistachios.

But, just like with proteins, where we need to go beyond the amount and look at its composition, when we look at fat we need to break down the fats into their type. See Chapter 2 for a detailed discussion of the fats.

In the common tree nuts, we find that . . .

- Almonds, cashews, hazelnuts, macadamias, pecans, and pistachios are high in monounsaturated fats.

- Pine nuts and walnuts are high in polyunsaturated fats.

- Brazil nuts have about the same amount of mono- and polyunsaturated fats.

- Walnuts have omega-3 fats, similar to those found in fish like salmon.

FIBER—A GIFT ONLY PLANT FOODS CAN GIVE

Carbohydrates are the body's primary energy source. The carbohydrate content of nuts varies from about 10 grams per ounce (about 35 percent) in cashew nuts to about 2 to 3 grams per ounce (10 percent) in Brazil nuts.

Most Americans consume too many refined carbohydrates, such as sugars and products made with white flour, and not enough unrefined carbohydrates. Unrefined carbohydrates such as fiber should compose most of one's diet. Most Americans consume about 12 grams of fiber per day, but should be consuming from 40 to 60 grams per day. Dietary fiber ranges from about 3 grams per ounce (about 11 percent) in almonds and pistachios to about 1 gram per ounce (about 3 percent) in cashews.

Nutrition, like medicine, is an ever-evolving science. It wasn't until the 1970s that fiber appeared on the horizon of nutritional science. Two now-famous British physicians, Hugh Trowell and Dennis Burkitt, came back from Uganda, Africa—then a part of the British Commonwealth—impressed by the fact that in their hospital, the native Ugandans eating a high-fiber, plant-based diet had hardly any of the diseases of the colon and heart that the local English residents had. They focused on fiber as the reason for this phenomenon, and we know now that they were right.

Fiber, found only in plant foods, alters the way fats affect us in two major ways. First, certain types of fiber lower cholesterol, and this alters the way fats affect our body. Second, some fibers help maintain a healthy digestive system, which results in regular bowel movements and easy elimination. This is protective against such diseases as colon cancer. One reason for this protective property is that when the diet is high in fiber, less time is taken by food residues and other by-products of digestion to move out of the body, quickly eliminating possible harmful compounds. Another reason is that fiber prevents the bowel from becoming alkaline, a condition some scientists think may open the way to some forms of bowel cancer. And fiber helps prevent those painful pouches in the colon called diverticula, commonly found during autopsies of people eating low-fiber, refined-food Western diets.

What's just as exciting is that with fiber comes many of the precious phytochemicals, another group of compounds totally overlooked by scientists until the late 1980s.

CALORIES

Carbohydrates, protein, and fat are the nutrients that supply energy to maintain life and make physical activity possible. The term "calorie" is used to measure energy in foods, and it is unfortunate that today we think of calories as something to keep as low as possible. Just like anything else in the diet, you want the right amount: not too little, not too much. But, above all, you want energy foods that satisfy you so you are less tempted to overeat. Calories in an ounce of nuts range from about 160 for cashews and pistachios, 165 for almonds, 180 for walnuts and hazelnuts, 190 for Brazil nuts and pecans, to about 200 for macadamias.

The key to better health is to obtain as many of your calories as possible from natural foods and plant foods, like nuts, that are rich in a multitude of precious compounds and fiber.

THE PHYTOCHEMICALS

Just when we thought we knew everything we needed to know about nutrition and health, a long list of compounds that we now call phytochemicals appeared on the horizon. As *phyto* means *plant* in the Greek language, phytochemical is a general name that could apply to all compounds in plants, but in recent years, it has been used in nutrition. There are thousands of precious compounds in foods, some of them soluble in water, some soluble in oils. In the good oils of nuts, we find different types of phytochemicals that are protective: the plant sterols, the antioxidants, and the saponins.

The Plant Sterols

Animal fats, such as we find in meats, poultry, and milk products, contain cholesterol. Instead of cholesterol, plant fats contain *plant sterols*, or phytosterols, which are slightly similar in their chemical structure to cholesterol, but instead of having bad effects on blood cholesterol, they actually help to lower it. Nuts and other unrefined plant foods are good sources of plant sterols. As these sterols are soluble in fat and not in water, we find more of them in plant foods that contain a reasonable amount of oils. Beyond cholesterol, some new research is showing that plant sterols have a protective effect against colon cancer. Plant sterols are another reason to consume a reasonable amount of seeds and other foods that supply good fat in an unrefined form.

The Antioxidants

Entire books have been written about antioxidants. They are compounds that nature placed in foods to protect fats from spoilage—rancidity—and that for centuries have been added to foods in the form of spices like sage, rosemary, and ginger to help preserve them. Unsaturated fats can spoil, so in nature they are rich in these protective antioxidants. Two types of chronic disease that antioxidants protect against are heart disease and cancer.

One group of major antioxidants in nuts is the tocopherols. The tocopherols are a group of several related compounds, most of which have vitamin-E activity. You could consider all the tocopherols like sisters and brothers—they all look very similar, but they have subtle differences in their chemical structure when you look closely at their molecules. Vitamin E is, chemically speaking, alpha-tocopherol and other sister tocopherols, such as beta-, delta-, and gamma-tocopherol. While alpha-tocopherol is, by far, the most potent as far as vitamin-E activity is concerned, the others not only have some vitamin-E activity, but are also good antioxidants. Gamma-tocopherol is such a powerful antioxidant that it is often used by the food industry as a natural antioxidant to preserve fats from spoilage. Recently, it has been found that higher intake of vitamin E is protective against heart disease.

Two other key phytochemicals found in nuts are quercetin and kaempferol. These powerful antioxidants seem to depress cancer growth. In laboratory experiments, Drs. John Miller and Penny Kris-Etherton of Pennsylvania State University have shown that both prostate and lung tumor growth was depressed by these two compounds. These compounds are also very powerful in preventing oxidation of cholesterol in the blood, and we know that this oxygen-damaged cholesterol is worse than non-oxidized cholesterol. But these are just a few powerful antioxidants in a thousand. Other powerful antioxidants are present in nuts and other plant foods.

Why are antioxidants so important? As much as oxygen is a key part of life, and we would soon die without it, in the complex biochemistry of the human body, molecules of oxygen can change to harmful compounds unless they are protected. These harmful compounds can damage a cell and open the door to cancer, or can damage cholesterol and make it much worse for us. Maybe that's why some Mediterranean societies have a low rate of heart disease: while they do not eat a low-fat diet, they consume plenty of fresh fruits and vegetables.

Large studies, such as one conducted by Dr. Michael Hertog in the Netherlands, have shown that high intakes of antioxidant-rich foods were connected with lower incidence of heart disease; and other studies have shown that antioxidants were related to lower rates of stomach cancer.

The Saponins

Saponins are complex molecules that are well known to pharmacologists for their often powerful biological effects. Some of them may work in concert with other compounds to lower blood cholesterol. The term *saponins* comes from the word soap, as they work in a similar way to soap. In the case of cholesterol, just think of saponins as having a cleansing action. Dr. David G. Oakenfull of the Division of Food Processing at CSIRO in New South Wales, Australia, proposes that some foods lower cholesterol partly because of their saponin content.

Drs. A.V. Rau and M.K. Sungh of the University of Toronto have shown that saponins have anticancer properties, and in 1995, they published a paper on their experiments with cancer cells. While that study was not done with nut saponins, it tells us that these substances have great disease-preventive potential.

Phytic Acid

Phytic acid, sometimes referred to as *phytate*, is present in the fibrous portion of plant foods and has been found to be protective against colon cancer, one of the most common cancers in industrialized countries, except for lung cancer in smokers. Phytates are fairly high in content in nuts, adding to their protective properties. Some scientists believe that it is compounds like phytates that make natural, high-fiber foods so protective against chronic diseases, as phytates normally go together with fiber. Phytates range in nuts from about 0.4 to 1 percent.

FOLIC ACID

Folic acid is one of the B vitamins and is often low in American diets. Nuts are good sources of folic acid. A component of blood nobody talked very much about until recently is the amino acid homocysteine. High levels of homocysteine in the blood go together with increased risk of heart disease. Folic acid—a vitamin that is better known for its function in making possible proper reproduction of red blood cells and other cells in the body—lowers homocysteine levels.

Folic acid ranges from about 16 to 20 micrograms per ounce in almonds, cashews, hazelnuts, pistachios and walnuts, to 11 micrograms in pecans and 5 in Brazil nuts and macadamias.

VITAMIN E AND TOCOPHEROLS

If I wanted to pick one key vitamin supplied by nuts, it would have to be vitamin E. Vitamin E is not only a vitamin, it is a powerful antioxidant, as well, and part of a very large family of compounds, called the tocopherols. All tocopherols are powerful antioxidants.

Some nuts have a large amount of alpha- and little gamma-tocopherol and others have large amounts of gamma- and little alpha-tocopherol. As both groups of tocopherols are extremely valuable, the wise choice is to eat a variety of nuts to obtain adequate amounts of both groups. For example, almonds and hazelnuts, which are high in alpha-tocopherol, go well with pecans or walnuts, which are high in gamma-tocopherol.

The minor tocopherols, called beta-tocopherol and delta-tocopherol, are present in very small amounts. Though they are protective and perform many of the same functions as the other tocopherols, we do not know too much about their specific functions. For the present, let's keep them in mind and part of the powerfully protective tocopherol family.

MINERALS

There are several minerals that are important for good health present in high amounts in nuts. Minerals that are high in content in nuts include potassium, copper, magnesium, and calcium.

Potassium and Sodium

Potassium is known to help to control blood pressure and is a key mineral for muscle and nerve function. Nuts are good sources of potassium and, if unsalted, very low in sodium, making them a good way to increase the potassium content of your diet without raising the sodium. Potassium content ranges from about 300 milligrams in an ounce of pistachios, to about 130 milligrams in an ounce of pecans and macadamias. Sodium is so low in unsalted nuts—a few milligrams, never more than 5 milligrams, per ounce—which means from a nutritional point of view that it is practically absent. Sodium intakes, even on low sodium diets, are measured in grams, that is, thousands of milligrams.

Magnesium and Calcium

Magnesium deficiency is associated with increased risk of heart disease. Calcium plays many major roles in the body. It not only builds bones, but it is also needed for the blood coagulation process, blood pressure regulation, muscle and nerve function, and many other life processes.

Nuts are good sources of magnesium. Its content ranges from 75 to 80 milligrams in an ounce of almonds, cashews, and hazelnuts, to about 35 milligrams in an ounce of pecans and macadamias.

Calcium is typically lower in seeds than magnesium and ranges from 75 milligrams in almonds, to about 10 milligrams in cashews and pecans.

Selenium

As selenium is not essential to proper plant growth, its content in a food depends on its presence or absence in the soil in which the food was grown. Selenium is a powerful antioxidant that has some properties similar to vitamin E. Many studies have shown a possible relationship between low selenium intake and a higher risk of cancer. In regions of China with soils extremely deficient in selenium, Keshan disease—a major heart malformation in infants—was a major health problem, until the government began to distribute selenium tablets to the population. The only nut truly rich in selenium is the Brazil nut, which grows in the tropical forest of Brazil, followed by the cashew nut when grown in the right soil.

Some Key Trace Minerals

There are two groups of minerals—those needed by the body in larger amounts, called major minerals, and those needed in smaller amounts, called trace minerals. Though trace minerals are only required in small amounts, they are vital to the proper functioning of the body. Nuts are good sources of many of them, such as copper, manganese, and zinc. For copper, cashews and hazelnuts are the stars; for manganese, the most important nuts are almonds and pecans; and for zinc, cashews and pecans.

Dr. Leslie Klevay of the Agricultural Research Service of the Human Nutrition Research Center of the United States Department of Agriculture (USDA) in North Dakota, considers copper to be a crucial mineral in heart disease prevention, as its deficiency has been associated with abnormal electrocardiogram readings (ECGs, the record of the electrical activity of the heart, producing its contractions), high blood cholesterol levels, and high blood pressure.

Table 3.1 shows the amount of some minerals in milligrams in 100 grams of nuts, and, again, we see how each nut complements the others nutritionally.

PUTTING IT ALL TOGETHER

Let's now go back to fats. By now we should realize that plant fats play a role in a healthy diet as long as we keep in mind that we must avoid highly purified fats. Eat nuts, avocados, and seeds to

Table 3.1. Some Minerals Present in Nuts (per 100 grams)

	Magnesium	Calcium	Potassium	Copper	Manganese	Zinc
Almonds	296 mg	266 mg	732 mg	1.0 mg	2.3 mg	3.0 mg
Brazil nuts	410 mg	170 mg	660 mg	1.8 mg	1.2 mg	4.2 mg
Cashews	260 mg	45 mg	663 mg	2.2 mg	1.0 mg	5.6 mg
Hazelnuts	285 mg	188 mg	680 mg	1.5 mg	2.0 mg	2.5 mg
Macadamias	115 mg	70 mg	370 mg	0.3 mg	4.1 mg	1.7 mg
Pecans	128 mg	70 mg	392 mg	1.2 mg	4.5 mg	5.5 mg
Pine nuts	270 mg	11 mg	520 mg	1.1 mg	4.6 mg	5.3 mg
Pistachios	158 mg	135 mg	1,100 mg	1.2 mg	1.2 mg	1.3 mg
Walnuts	170 mg	95 mg	500 mg	1.4 mg	3.0 mg	2.7 mg

obtain your fat, and when you use oils, be sure they are unrefined. When I refer to fats in the diet, I am referring to *natural* fats, with all their protective compounds.

Scientists are just beginning to understand the way plant proteins, fiber, phytochemicals, and fats work together. Even so, it's easy to see that much of the confusion about the role of fats comes from our frequent attempt to put that compound on the stand and have a jury judge them as though they lived a life of their own. These poor fats in that courtroom are in tears, unjustly condemned and removed from our diet, together with all the other great compounds they carry with them. Let's reach out to them and do them justice.

The key point to remember is that you must take all that I have said in the context of *whole, natural, higher-fat foods from plants,* such as nuts, many seeds, avocados, and olives, which contain many other precious substances that can alter the way these fats affect us. Do not extrapolate all this to apply to highly purified fat products.

If, for whatever reason, you want to be on a very low-fat diet, remember that a few nuts a week will add many valuable nutrients to your diet, will help you to feel satisfied, and will hardly alter the amount of fat in your diet—in fact, they will add the very important good fats to your diet, which you will probably be missing if you are cutting fat from your diet. Reach for a few nuts in place of saturated fat sources whenever your body craves some fat.

As we look back at this chapter, it's clear that nuts have many great nutrients in common, and that each nut has something special and different to offer. Two key lessons in good nutrition emerge from what we have just learned:

- No matter how great tree nuts and others seeds are, we need to combine them with other foods.

- Even though tree nuts have many similarities, we may gain by consuming more than one nut as each one has its own star nutrients.

Read Chapter 18 to learn about other foods that, when combined with nuts, result in a good, sound, disease-prevention diet.

In the next chapter, you will learn that clinical research with nuts of different types confirms that they play a crucial role in a healthy diet. And this research also lends additional support to the concept that plant fats, at a reasonable level, are not only acceptable but are beneficial for the majority of the population.

4

Nuts in Disease Prevention

One way we study the effects of foods and nutrients on health is to take a large population and follow it for many years, finding out what they eat or don't eat, what are their major chronic diseases (like cancer and heart disease), and what causes their death. This is sometimes called an *epidemiological* or *population* study. Another way is to take a group of people and feed them a certain food or diet, comparing this to different foods or diets under more or less controlled conditions. This latter type of research is usually called a *clinical* or *intervention* study. Often a large population study is followed by an intervention study to try to confirm the results of the population study. Finally, observations may be made that may not be considered at the same level of reliability as a properly designed study, but when scrutinized by a scientist can add to our knowledge of the benefits or harmfulness of various foods or substances. Let's look at nuts and their effects on our health using both types of research methods.

NUTS AND HEART DISEASE

Many of the studies that follow are about prevention of heart disease. Why? Because heart disease is the number-one killer in the United States and most industrialized countries. In developing countries, as Western foods are introduced to the diet, heart disease goes up. Heart disease far outweighs diabetes, accidents, and even cancer as a cause of death in the United States. This makes heart disease prevention a number-one priority.

It is now well established that high levels of blood cholesterol mean greater risk of heart disease. In fact, the higher one's blood cholesterol level, the more likely one is to die as a result of heart disease. It's logical that we need foods that help to keep blood cholesterol levels low.

The Adventist Health Study

Dr. Gary Fraser, professor of Medicine and Epidemiology, and director of the Center for Health Research in the School of Public Health at Loma Linda University in Loma Linda, California, talks about the study he carried out with Dr. Joan Sabaté and other researchers at Loma Linda, with over 34,000 people:

> *We call the study The Adventist Health Study. In 1974 through 1975 we identified about 34,000—34,192 to be exact—California Seventh-Day Adventists. The reason that we chose these people is that their dietary habits are interesting; about half of them eat very little or no meat at all, and they use a variety of other foods more so than the typical American. One of the differences is somewhat more of a focus on nuts, which means that we could investigate that food with much more power and accuracy than perhaps many other studies. After we identified these people in 1974 through 1975, we followed them, looking for clinical problems, such as heart attacks and cancers, for six years, through 1982, and then for another six or seven years just following for causes of death.*
>
> *We had designed a very detailed questionnaire, and these people had sufficient interest and enthusiasm for the project because they completed this questionnaire and gave us a lot of good information by mail as to what their dietary habits were, what their health history was, how they exercised, and so forth. Then about every year, we would send them a questionnaire*

that asked them if they had been hospitalized in the last twelve months and, if so, where. At the time, we had about 800 hospitals within California and probably about another 1,000 outside of California where we had to either go to their medical records rooms, if they were in California, or communicate by mail with hospitals outside of California to check and see if the hospitalization was for a heart attack. More than that, we had our study representatives within California use microfilm cameras, and we filmed all of the electrocardiograms showing us how healthy or unhealthy their hearts were. We made copies of all the blood tests that related to heart health, copies of the doctors' histories and then used some standardized coding formulas to enter all this data in our databases. When we put together all this information, it gave us good evidence whether they had had a heart attack or not. We did the same for cancer, using the slides from medical records to make that diagnosis.

When we designed the study we had only a small interest in nuts. We knew they were fatty foods, and no one had really investigated them before, or we didn't have strong opinions about their role in the diet. So we had only one question [relating to nuts], "How many times per day, per week, per month do you eat nuts of any kind?" We had a rating of about eight different possibilities of the frequency of consuming nuts that we got from these 34,000 people, and later we were able to relate that to their risk of the heart attack—either a fatal one resulting in death or nonfatal.

To our surprise, we found that the people who ate nuts frequently, four to five times each week, as compared with people who hardly ate nuts, had a much lower risk of heart attack, whether fatal or nonfatal.

The participants in that study completed a detailed twenty-four-hour recall of all the foods they ate and did this for five separate days over a period of some months. We also asked, not only about frequency, but [about] how many nuts they normally consumed. It turned out that, on average, it was about one-and-one-half to two ounces, which is a moderate-sized handful. If we wanted to apply this to recommend something to the general population, my suggestion would be one to two ounces, three to four times a week.

Why are nuts protective against heart disease? Is it the type of fat, the fiber, the many phytochemicals, or the vitamin E? [These questions are] still open to research, but I think it's probably a combination of several factors for this reason: There is now a good amount of evidence that at least several of the nuts can lower blood cholesterol as compared to other more typical fats in the diet, and yet the degree of lowering—low to substantial—is not really enough to account for a 50-percent lowering of heart disease risk that we have documented in our study. It seems there's probably something else going on in there. Possibly things like vitamin E and other phytochemicals with their antioxidant potential may play a key role.

Dr. Leslie Klevay of the USDA in North Dakota has suggested that the protective effect of nuts found in the Loma Linda study may be due to the copper content of nuts, a mineral often deficient in the American diet.

The Iowa Women's Study

Dr. Larry Kushi, associate professor in the Division of Epidemiology in the School of Public Health at the University of Minnesota in Minneapolis, is one of the directors of the large Iowa Women's Study, a study in which a large number of women—about 38,000—has been followed for many years. Kushi states:

The more frequently the women ate nuts, the lower their heart-disease risk. This was true even when the nut consumption was only a few times a week. And if you actually compare our results with the Seventh-Day Adventist Study, they seem to correspond quite well. The Seventh-Day Adventists do have a larger proportion of the population with a somewhat higher intake of nuts, but, still, over the same range, we seem to see a similar sort of relationship. Dr. Walter Willett of Harvard has done the same analysis in the Nurses' Study, and they see the same thing: a decreased risk with nut consumption.

My Studies

As I learned of the Loma Linda study in the 1980s, I felt the time had come to do some clinical studies on nuts and some of the risk factors for heart disease, like high blood cholesterol. Inspired by Fraser and his colleagues, I did two major studies with almonds in the Health Research and Studies Center together with other researchers. At that time, olive oil was also coming to the forefront of nutrition as a beneficial oil, and stories were often found in newspapers of Mediterranean people consuming olive oil and nuts in diets high in plant foods.

We did two major studies, and in both studies we fed about three ounces of almonds each day to the subjects. The first study was a nine-week study using raw almonds, some whole and unblanched (with their skins on) and some ground so that the subjects could sprinkle them on cereals, salads, and other foods or use them as part of a prepared dish. This large amount of almonds became the primary source of fat in the diet, with almond oil as the only permitted vegetable oil or fat. Of the twenty-seven hypercholesterolemic (having high blood-cholesterol levels) adult males and females who completed the study, blood cholesterol was reduced in three weeks by 10 percent and low-density-lipoprotein (LDL) cholesterol (the so-called "bad" cholesterol) was reduced by 12 percent, with no change in high-density-lipoprotein (HDL) cholesterol (the "good" cholesterol) or triglycerides. These levels were maintained over the nine weeks of the study. There was no significant change in body weight.

Following this study, we wanted to compare the effect of almonds—with their beautiful complexity of good fats, plant proteins, phytochemicals, fiber, and carbohydrates—to two different diets. One of the other diets had the same type of fat in the form of olive oil, which we know is a good monounsaturated oil similar to almond oil, along with animal protein from cottage cheese and yogurt. The other control diet was based on saturated fat from cheese—which, as far as we know, does not lower blood cholesterol—and the animal protein of cheese. We matched the amount of protein in the almonds to the animal protein in the other two diets and added some cereal fiber to match the amount of fiber.

After the subjects ate these three different diets for four weeks, almonds caused a very meaningful lowering of both blood cholesterol (8 percent) and LDL cholesterol (14 percent), while, again, there was no decrease in the good HDL cholesterol. The olive oil group did not do so well, and the blood-cholesterol lowering was very minor. The most likely reason—which supports the importance of all the components of the diet working together in the control of cholesterol—is that animal protein was used—cottage cheese and yogurt—rather than the plant protein present in the almond. The cheese group, as expected, did not experience any lowering of cholesterol.

The results of this study remind us that we cannot take an isolated oil, be it olive oil or a nut oil, and expect it to work independently of the other components of the diet. Take olive oil as part of a good plant-based Mediterranean diet: we could not expect the same results on a diet high in meat, poultry, and dairy products and low in grains, beans, fruits, vegetables, and nuts— the results would be quite different.

Almonds are typical monounsaturated-fat nuts, but so are cashews, hazelnuts, macadamias, pistachios, and pecans. Though promising studies on some of these nuts and their effects on blood cholesterol are in progress, they have not yet been clinically studied as extensively as almonds; however, we may expect that these nuts also have beneficial effects on blood cholesterol.

Macadamia Nut Studies

In Australia, Dr. David M. Colquhoun and his associates at the University of Queensland compared a diet high in macadamia nuts—the Australian native nut—to a diet high in carbohydrates. They found both diets effective in lowering total blood cholesterol by about 7 percent and LDL cholesterol by about 11 percent. HDL cholesterol was lowered by the high-carbohydrate diet, but not by the macadamia nut diet.

Dr. David Curb at the University of Hawaii looked at a different aspect of the blood-cholesterol story. He wanted to determine the effect of feeding macadamia nuts to people with fairly normal cholesterol, who were not in need of lowering their blood-cholesterol levels. Curb compared an American Heart Association diet, fairly low in fat (30-percent calories from fat), with a typical American diet (37-percent calories from fat) and a macadamia-nut diet (also with 37-percent calories from fat, but with most of the fat coming from macadamia nuts). The macadamia-nut diet lowered blood cholesterol even in these normal subjects from about 200 to 191 milligrams, and this change was similar to that of the lower-fat diet. What was the reason? Very likely, the cause was the lower saturated fat in both diets resulting from lower intake of higher fat—usually saturated fat—animal products.

The Loma Linda Walnut Study

Dr. Joan Sabaté, associate professor of Nutrition, Epidemiology and Biology in the Schools of Public Health and Medicine at Loma Linda University, conducted a study on the effects of walnuts on heart disease. Below, he explains this study.

After working with a large population study that showed that frequency of nut consumption lowered the risk of heart disease, I became interested in knowing through what mechanism that could be. I thought about a type of a study that tested one nut at a time, and I studied walnuts to test the effect of walnuts on the blood cholesterol. To do so, I selected healthy subjects that had normal cholesterol—they were perfectly healthy and relatively young—and I asked if they would be willing to come to my research kitchen for two months and consume the meals that I would prepare for them. Eighteen did accept this invitation and were fed two diets. All subjects were fed the two diets but in different order, and the two diets were: (1) a diet that contained two to three ounces of walnuts, which varied according to the caloric needs of the subjects and their weight and height; and (2) a healthy diet [that] nowadays is recommended for lowering cholesterol, which we call the American Heart Association Step-1 diet. So I did not compare a walnut diet with a traditional American diet that we know has room for improvement; I compared against a diet that is what physicians and health authorities recommend for lowering cholesterol.

As expected, while subjects were on this cholesterol-lowering diet, their cholesterol improved and went down. I would not say it was surprising, but it was quite interesting that while on the walnut diet, the same subjects' cholesterol decreased further—[total] blood cholesterol by 12 percent and LDL cholesterol, 16 percent. In short, being fed a diet high in walnuts, the subjects' cholesterol decreased more than [the cholesterol of] the same subjects being fed a diet that physicians recommend for lowering cholesterol.

The other interesting measurements we did in this study were of triglycerides [major fats in the blood], and they went down, although not significantly, and HDL cholesterol stayed pretty much stable. Just as important, the ratio of bad cholesterol (LDL cholesterol) to good cholesterol (HDL), a ratio that is highly predictive for the risk of heart disease, improved.

The subjects had to consume two to three ounces of walnuts daily. I prepared the meals for them, as I mentioned. It's not as if I gave them to the subjects and then sent them home; they came to the kitchen. So the walnuts were incorporated in several ways, because I did not want them to have a monotonous diet. One way was as a snack, which they had to eat in addition to [their meals]. We did other things, such as incorporating walnuts into pizza, into salad, into morning cereal. We ground walnuts with hamburgers, so instead of giving a full hamburger it was meat plus walnuts plus a little bit of flour, and made walnut patties. By the way, you can do walnut patties without meat at all, just with egg whites, walnuts, flour, and some seasoning. We incorporated walnuts also into selected dishes. Besides, walnuts are consumed in this country as part of baked goods, in breads, desserts or cakes, so we also incorporated this, and with pasta.

As walnuts are high in polyunsaturated fat, we measured the concentration of these fats in the blood. And we found a slight increase, not a dramatic increase, but a slight increase. There was about a 25-percent increase of the omega-3 fats, the kind you get by eating fish. Walnuts could be a good source of omega-3.

The Australian Study on Almonds and Walnuts

In Australia, Dr. Mavis Abbey and associates at CSIRO, Division of Human Nutrition in Adelaide, fed almonds, a typical monounsaturated nut, or walnuts, a polyunsaturated nut. Otherwise, the subjects were fed a similar, typical Australian diet. This nine-week study was different from the almond studies done at the Health Research and Studies Center, as the sixteen male subjects in the almond-walnut study had normal, rather then elevated, levels of blood cholesterol. These men, for three weeks, consumed a typical Australian diet with its typical fat composition. Some of the fat sources were then replaced for three weeks by almonds and for another three weeks by walnuts. With the raw almond supplementation, total blood cholesterol dropped by 7 percent and LDL cholesterol, by 10 percent; and with walnuts, total blood cholesterol dropped by 5 percent and LDL cholesterol, by 9 percent. In both cases, the good HDL cholesterol did not go down.

The Jerusalem Nutrition Study

Dr. Elliot Berry and his associates at the Hebrew University in Jerusalem examined the relationship between a diet high in polyunsaturated fats and a diet high in monounsaturated fats and heart disease as part of The Jerusalem Nutrition Study. This study was not exclusively a "nut" study, like the studies we have just reviewed, but nuts were an important part of the experimental diets, as the focus was on the fat composition of the diet. The subjects were twenty-six young university students from the Yeshiva Har Etzion College outside Jerusalem, who seemed ideal for such an experiment. At this college, students are required to attend school from early in the morning to late in the evening and to eat their meals at the college cafeteria. Dr. Berry devised a diet high in monounsaturated fats, including almonds, avocados, and olive oil; and a diet high in polyunsaturated fats, including walnuts, safflower oil, and soybean oil.

The group consuming the almond/high-monounsaturated-fat diet had an average decrease in total blood cholesterol of 10 percent and in LDL cholesterol of 14 percent. The walnut/high-polyunsaturated-fat diet group experienced a 16-percent reduction in total blood cholesterol and a 20-percent decrease in LDL cholesterol, with no reduction in high-density lipoprotein (HDL) cholesterol.

In another part of The Jerusalem Nutrition Study, students from the same college were assigned to either a high-mono diet, as just described—high in almonds, avocados, and olive oil—or a high-carbohydrate diet. The almond-mono diet resulted, again, in a total blood cholesterol reduction of about 8 percent and a 14-percent reduction of LDL cholesterol, again without significant changes in HDL cholesterol. The high-carbohydrate diet did not result in any changes in blood cholesterol. On the high almond-mono diet, cholesterol seemed to be more protected from damaging oxidation than on the high-carbohydrate diet.

My Studies on Tree Nuts as Part of Plant-Based Diets

At the Health Research and Studies Center, we went a step further and studied some real-life situations where mixed nuts, nut products, and seeds like sesame were fed as part of a healthy, vegetarian diet based on whole, unrefined, ancient foods, such as whole grains, dried fruits like raisins, and plenty of vegetables and fruits. For four weeks, the free-living subjects ate this Mediterranean-type diet, high in total and soluble fibers and monounsaturated fats. Sun-dried raisins, whole-grain raisin bread, almonds and almond butter, hazelnuts, walnuts, and other nuts, along with some sesame butter and some olive oil, were given to fifteen subjects with high blood cholesterol. The subjects' total blood cholesterol decreased by 8 percent and their LDL cholesterol decreased by 15 percent, with no significant changes in the good cholesterol.

Following the positive results of this study, we placed twelve nonsmoking, postmenopausal women on a low-fruit-and-vegetable, highly-refined-carbohydrate diet for four weeks. These women freely ate white bread, white rice, and meat and other animal products, but a minimum of fruits and vegetables. Tree nuts and dried fruits were excluded from this diet, which we called the *"depleting" diet*, and measurements were made at the end of this period. Afterwards, these subjects were placed on a diet high in fruits and vegetables, whole grains, and mixed nuts and seeds— the *"good" diet*. After four weeks on the "good" diet, there were major reductions of 13 percent in total cholesterol and 16 percent in LDL cholesterol. Again, as expected, when there was enough fat in the diet and the diet was based on unrefined carbohydrates, there was essentially no change in the good cholesterol.

As this was a diet high in protective antioxidants, we measured the levels of some protective enzymes in the blood cells and in the blood plasma—the clear portion of the blood in which the cells are suspended—and found that the need for these enzymes decreased. This probably meant that, because of the nuts, raisins, whole grains, green tea, and all the other good plant foods, the diet was so rich in antioxidants that the body needed less of its own defenses to protect its tissues from damage.

Nuts and Blood Clotting

The lower risk for heart disease we have seen in the large population studies may be due to decreased risk of abnormal blood clot formation. This kind of clot that forms inside an artery is called a thrombus, and if it clogs one of the arteries that feed the heart muscle—the coronary arteries—it will inevitably lead to a heart attack. Could it be that one way nuts prevent heart disease is by preventing this kind of problem?

One reason for this beneficial effect of nuts in preventing blood clotting could be the effect of nuts on platelets. Platelets are small particles present in blood that promote blood clotting. Aggregation, that is, clumping together, of platelets is a key process in making blood coagulation possible after an injury that causes bleeding. But abnormal, excessive aggregation of platelets can lead to problems.

NUTS AND CANCER

There is evidence that nuts may protect against cancer as well. Let's look at some studies that have explored this effect.

Cashews and Cancer

Dr. Bandaru Reddy, chief of the Division of Nutritional Carcinogenesis at the School of Public Health of the American Health
Foundation in Valhalla, New York, sees a correlation between the
intake of cashews and low incidence of colon cancer.

> *Cashew nuts are grown extensively in the southwestern part
> of India, and many Indians in that region and in several other
> parts of India eat a lot of cashews as a snack, sometimes raw,
> but mostly roasted. Throughout India, cashews are used in
> cooking, often as an important part of a recipe. There is an
> interesting potential health benefit: there appears to be an
> inverse relationship between the occurrence of cancer of the
> colon and cashew nuts' consumption in India. But we have to
> be somewhat cautious in interpreting these results, as [the
> incidence of] colon cancer in India is one of the lowest in the
> world. Still, cashews appear to have some protective effect.*

Nuts and Stomach Cancer

Stomach cancer is not a major killer in the United States and other
Western countries, but it is in Japan and other Asian countries. Drs.
Hoshiyama and Sasaba of Japan studied the relationship of diet
and smoking and drinking habits in Japan in 1992. While in this
study the main protective factors were fruits, vegetables, and sea-
weed, subjects who never ate nuts had a greater risk of stomach
cancer than subjects who ate them even a few times a month. This
should not be considered a nut study, but rather a study that
shows that nuts can be part of a good plant-based diet.

NUTS AND BLOOD PRESSURE

Nuts are good sources of potassium and magnesium, minerals that
are key in the control of blood pressure. The large DASH study—
the study of Dietary Approaches to Stop Hypertension—found
nuts to be a highly desirable part of the diet. As it is known that
populations eating vegetarian diets worldwide have lower blood

pressures, the DASH researchers tested diets high in various plant foods. Some of the key differences in the DASH diet are higher intakes of potassium, magnesium, and fiber—all nutrients found in high quantities in nuts. The results of the DASH study confirm that increasing plant food consumption helps to control blood pressure.

Plant-based diets have much more potassium than sodium, and unsalted nuts are high in potassium and extremely low in sodium—you could call unsalted nuts sodium-free—one reason unsalted nuts should be considered a key part of blood-pressure control. It is possible that arginine, too, may play a role in the blood-pressure-lowering effect of nuts, due to its effect of relaxing blood vessels.

Next, in Part Two, we will take a close look at the individual nuts, including their history, lore, and health benefits.

PART TWO

Tree Nuts
of the World

5

Nuts on Every Continent

ature in her wisdom has placed a large number of trees producing edible nuts on every continent that is not covered by ice, so that the continent's natives—in the days when transportation was slow and often difficult, and the food they ate was the food they found or grew in their own region— would be able to have these precious seeds. That nut trees were found all over the world is another reminder of how nature considered nuts a very valuable food. As the civilizations evolved and transportation became less and less primitive, nut trees moved across vast plains and large oceans to reach other continents.

Some of these tree nuts have been, and are, used as energy and protein foods; others, such as nutmeg, have unique characteristics and are used as spices; and others, like the acorn from oaks, have faded into obscurity as better-tasting nuts moved in from other regions. Some nuts, like Brazil nuts, did not adapt well when people tried to plant them outside of their native habitats.

In the chapters that follow we'll explore in greater depth the history of the common tree nuts.

HOW NUTS TRAVELED TO NEW REGIONS

Major changes occurred when people learned to farm, grow grains, and tame animals for meat, milk, and egg production. As millennia passed, the quest for food in a forest by primitive people was slowly being replaced more and more by farming, which then became the major source of food for humanity. Nuts not only continued to be a key part of the diet, but as nut trees became cultivated rather than wild, it became easier to have nuts available. That nuts were held in high esteem throughout history is shown by how many types of nuts moved across continents to be cultivated away from their native habitats.

As people began to move from some regions of the earth to other distant ones, the goodness of nuts fascinated early travelers and writers. From the Persian region to China, from Europe to the Americas, from Brazil to India, nuts and nut trees found their way around the world. As people began to add nuts to their diet, they very likely found them to be health- and energy-giving and easy to keep without spoilage for prolonged periods, just like pre-agricultural societies did in the age of hunter-gatherers.

The movement of nuts across oceans and continents was helped by the interests of leaders of earlier centuries. One of them, Thomas Jefferson, while U.S. minister to France, became fascinated by the large cultivation of various nuts in France and Italy. He traveled through the regions—a major effort in the days when travel was only by horse-drawn carriage—and studied the cultivation of the major typical nuts of these regions: almonds, pistachios, and walnuts. Jefferson was hoping that these nuts could be grown in the then newly formed United States, to add to the local pecans and pine nuts.

THE MAJOR TREE NUTS

In the chapters that follow, we'll learn more about nine of the major tree nuts common today: almonds, Brazil nuts, cashews, hazelnuts, macadamias, pecans, pine nuts, pistachios, and walnuts. While in Chapter 3 we compared all the common nuts for their nutritional goodness, in the following chapters we'll focus on the history, lore, and what is special about each nut. The uses of nuts in today's diets, and suggestions for ultimate diets using nuts, will be found in Chapters 16 and 17.

6

The Almond— Queen of the Rose Family

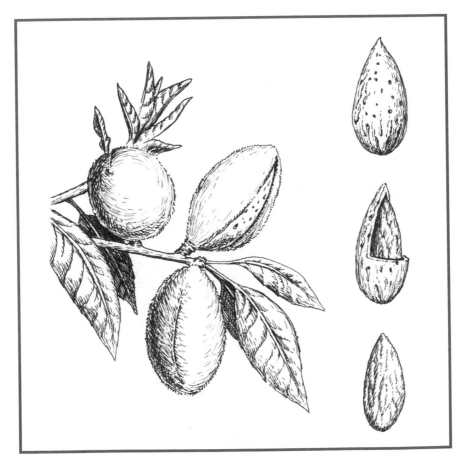

A lmonds belong to the rose family, the *Rosaceae*, and the almond has been called the queen of the rose family. Its Latin name, *Prunus dulcis*, implies sweetness (*dulcis* means sweet). You may also find another Latin name for the almond, *Prunus amygdalus*. The fruits of the rose family are many and include apples, pears, prunes, and apricots. If you crack the stone of an apricot, you'll find a bitter nut inside that looks like an almond and is edible, reminding us that the apricot is a close relative of the almond, and some bitter varieties of almonds—*Prunus amara*—not commonly used, taste like apricot seeds.

In Southern Mediterranean countries, almonds are often grown together with olives, and both trees are considered sacred in the minds of many of the local peasants.

FROM ASIA TO THE WORLD

The almond is native to Asia. The almond traveled early in history, making it difficult to pinpoint a region of origin. "Recent discoveries in the highlands of eastern Turkey," Dr. Michael Rosenburg of the University of Delaware tells us, "indicate the existence there already 10,000 years ago of fully settled village societies with economies dependent on the intensive exploitation of almonds and pistachios."

The Phoenicians—members of an ancient civilization of Southwest Asia—lived in what is today Syria and Lebanon—and traveled the Mediterranean Sea extensively in the twelfth century B.C. They took many of their native foods with them to other countries and are the ones who most likely introduced the almond to various Mediterranean countries like Greece, Italy, Spain, and France. The almond was known to the Hebrews centuries before Christ, and the almond tree is mentioned in the Book of Genesis many times. And again the almond is mentioned in Jeremiah, "The word of the Lord came to me: 'What do you see, Jeremiah?' 'I see the branch of an almond tree,' I replied." (Jeremiah 1:11).

Later, the almond traveled to Germany, and much later, in the seventeenth century, almonds reached England and the Americas. Missionaries traveling to California from Mexico and Spain to establish the California missions brought the almond to California.

But it was only in the mid-nineteenth century, about 1843, that almonds began to be grown commercially in California from trees brought from the east coast of the United States. Today California, together with Mediterranean countries like Italy, is one of the largest producers of almonds.

LORE AND ANCIENT USES OF ALMONDS

The use of almonds in folk remedies was very popular over the centuries. Some historians believe that cooks of royal families in medieval times—that period in European history between antiquity and the Renaissance from the fifth to the fifteenth century—added almonds to many dishes as they seemed to help the over-indulging royalty to better digest their heavy meat dishes.

Almonds were a key part of recipes in medieval Mediterranean countries from France to Italy, Spain, and Greece. John Heinerman writes in his *Encyclopedia of Nuts, Berries and Seeds:* "An inventory of the household goods of the Queen of France in 1372 listed only twenty pounds of sugar—but included over five hundred pounds of almonds."

Taillevent was a fourteenth-century (1312–1395) master chef to the French royalty, and his book *Le Viandier* could probably be considered the first classic cookbook. He had risen at age fourteen from kitchen boy—a very lowly position—to cook and was given a house for his services. He wrote about using almonds, both ground and whole, as a major part of chicken recipes. Jean-Francois Revel, in his 1982 book *Culture and Cuisine*, describes how Taillevent cooked capon in boiling water, removed the white meat, ground almonds and put it through a sieve, boiled this again, strained it, boiled it to thicken it, added some fried almonds and, finally, added sugar. This may be a strange mixture for our modern tastes, but it is an indication of how almonds were key ingredients of many recipes of that era. Could it be that the almond—or perhaps other nuts available in Europe in those days, such as hazelnuts, pine nuts, pistachios, or walnuts—made this amazing dish "healthier" and easier on the digestive system?

Almond milk was widely used for flavoring and thickening in many English recipes in medieval times. Lorna Sass, in her *To the*

King's Taste, tells us that "One of the most popular ingredients in medieval cooking, almond milk, was so commonly known that few cooks bothered to write the recipe down." She quotes a 1542 recipe for almond milk to " . . . mollyfe [mollify] the belly." Almond and walnut milks were still commonly used in cooking in Europe until the beginning of the nineteenth century.

In another book, *Curye on Inglysch*, Constance Hieatt and Sharon Butler, in 1985, brought back to life original recipes published in the fourteenth century. When we translate the recipes written in old English, we find almond and pine nut milks widely used. These two were very common nuts in England in those days and, together with walnuts and pistachios, were part of many other dishes.

In one recipe from *Curye on Inglysch*, for a main dish where chicken is cooked in broth—a very common way of cooking in earlier centuries in Europe and even today—blanched almond milk was combined with ginger and chicken cut up into morsels, and this mixture was boiled and served. In another recipe made with the breast meat of capon—a castrated male chicken so treated to improve the taste of its flesh—almond milk was boiled with rice and then the capon flesh was cooked in this broth. In some recipes, we find "crem," a thick cream of almond milk curdled with vinegar, often used with pork and chicken dishes. Boiled almond milk also was added to onion soups and other soups.

In the Europe of aristocracy and royalty of past centuries we find that nuts such as almonds, pine nuts, hazelnuts, pistachios, and walnuts were the nuts commonly available in Europe in medieval times. The concept that nuts made meat and chicken dishes healthier appears to have been well accepted. Later, we'll see that the Queen of Sheba in ancient times considered pistachio nuts a precious food, probably because they made her Court healthier.

That nuts aided digestion wasn't just ancient lore. It is probably true, as the Italian official list of medications in 1929 listed *Acqua di mandorle amare* (water of bitter almonds), in which almonds were extracted with alcohol and water and then the liquid portion distilled to produce a clear liquid that was recommended as an antispasmodic for convulsive cough and stomach problems. A similar preparation made with sweet almonds was used as an aid to digestion and to normalize bowel function.

According to Mary Reed, in her book *Fruits & Nuts in Symbolism & Celebration*, almonds over the centuries have been considered a sign of fertility, happiness, romance, good health, and fortune. The Romans, for example, showered newlyweds with almonds.

ALMOND MILK FOR ANCIENT CHINESE INFANTS

As China was a nonpastoral society, dairy milks were not part of the normal diet. The Chinese—remember that the Chinese had found green and black teas to be beneficial beverages hundreds of years before we discovered that they were high in antioxidants— held almond milk in such high esteem that Reay Tannahill, in her *Food in History* says: " . . . almond milk had a high nutritional reputation and was poured down the throats of privileged infants in astonishing quantities."

THE NUTRITIONAL PROPERTIES OF ALMONDS

The almonds, together with cashews, hazelnuts, macadamias, pecans, and pistachios, belong to the group of nuts that are high in monounsaturated fat. Almonds are also among the nuts highest in dietary fiber (more than 3 grams in an ounce), which is important for good digestive function and satiety and perhaps for blood cholesterol control, and in plant sterols (one ounce of almonds contains about 75 milligrams). And they are highest in calcium (75 milligrams in an ounce). They are good sources of protein (5.6 grams per ounce) and of folic acid (about 18 micrograms per ounce).

Almonds are high in alpha-tocopherol, with over 6.5 milligrams in an ounce. There is about .5 milligram of gamma-tocopherol and traces of beta-tocopherol in an ounce of almonds. An ounce of almonds also contains about 90 milligrams of magnesium and about 220 milligrams of potassium.

7

Brazil Nuts— The Rain Forest Nuts

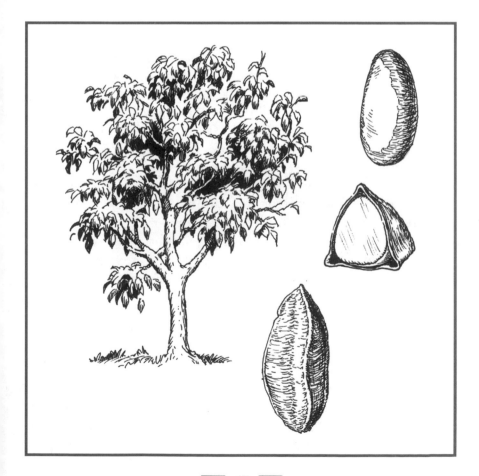

While so many of the other tree nuts have traveled successfully to other regions, the Brazil nut (*Bertholletia myrtaceae or excelsa*), native to the Amazon region—in fact, it has been called the Amazon nut—seems to be so much in love with the local environment that it has resisted any attempt to successfully grow it in other regions of the world.

Brazil nut trees are very large—75 to 150 feet high, with trunks that often measure ten feet in diameter—and form large, picturesque forests along the Amazon and Rio Grande rivers in South America. The nuts grow inside a pod, and inside the pod, the nuts are arranged in a way similar to the segments of an orange. This wild tree seems to bear about the same amount of nuts every year, while the yield of some cultivated nuts, like the almond, varies from year to year. The French call Brazil nuts *American chestnuts.*

THE NUTRITIONAL PROPERTIES OF THE BRAZIL NUT

As the selenium content of a food depends on the presence of selenium in the soil in which it is grown—selenium is not needed for plant growth and development—the Brazil nut is blessed by the Amazon soil in the tropics, soil that is extremely rich in selenium. While other common nuts contain just traces of selenium (4 to 40 micrograms in 100 grams), Brazil nuts contain from 230 to 5,300 micrograms in 100 grams, depending on the soil in Brazil where they grew, with an average of 1,530 micrograms in 100 grams. Don't forget that a few micrograms of many substances are often all we need for a protective action. Remember that selenium is a mineral with powerful antioxidant properties. It is essential to health and may help prevent some types of cancer. Selenium deficiency in China has led to heart malformations in infants.

The Brazil nut is unique in many ways. It is one of the few common nuts that has about the same amount of mono- and poly-unsaturated fats. One ounce of Brazil nuts contains about 4 grams of protein, 1.5 grams of fiber, about 1.5 micrograms of folic acid, 50 milligrams of calcium, and about 180 milligrams of potassium. Finally, Brazil nuts are a great source of gamma-tocopherol (almost 4 milligrams per ounce), a powerful antioxidant and relative of vitamin E. They have 2 milligrams of alpha-tocopherol and about .05 milligram of beta- and delta-tocopherol in an ounce.

8

Cashew Nuts—
The Nuts of
Ayurvedic Medicine

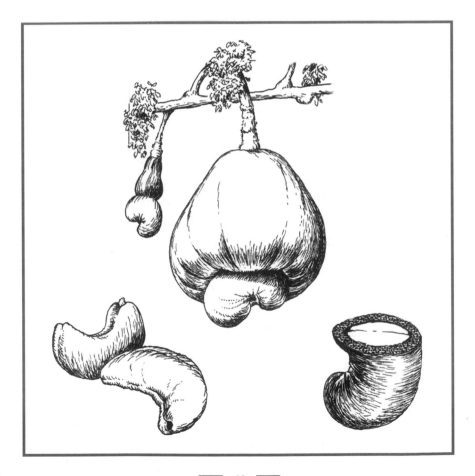

Cashews (*Anarcardium occidentale*) are native to Brazil, like the Brazil nut. Cashews were given their botanical name because they are heart-shaped (-cardium). Both the Spanish and Italian names for cashews include the root *cardio* or *cardo*, for heart. The cashew tree belongs to the same family as the pistachio and is a fast-growing, evergreen perennial. It loves the tropics and in tropical heat can grow to heights of forty or fifty feet.

The cashew fruit has two distinct parts: the fleshy pear-shaped stalk or stem known as the *cashew apple*, two to four inches in length, and the heart-shaped—sometimes called kidney-shaped—nut, the true fruit, about an inch in length, that is attached to the lower end of the apple. The nut, like other nuts, contains the edible kernel. The "apple" is not only edible but delicious and rich in vitamin C, but it is practically unknown outside of regions where cashew trees grow, as are its products like cashew apple wine.

FROM BRAZIL TO ASIA AND AFRICA

Cashew nuts, unlike the Brazil nut, have traveled well away from Brazil, and today India is one of the major producers of cashews, so much so that some people think that cashews are native to India. The cashew tree likes the jungle and the tropics and, contrary to its tropical Brazilian sister the Brazil nut, the cashew loves to travel. In 1558, Thevet, a French naturalist, visited the territory of Maranhao in Northern Brazil and observed the natives harvesting and eating cashews. By 1590, cashews had been introduced to India, to Mozambique in East Africa, and to other tropical regions by early Portuguese missionaries and seamen.

HARVESTING CASHEWS

The ripe cashew apples are allowed to fall to the ground. They are then gathered, and the nuts are sun-dried for two days. But don't expect to go to the store to buy cashew nuts in their shells as you would buy most other nuts to crack at home. The cashew kernel is protected by a double shell with the space between shells filled by a resinous liquid that has many industrial uses. In India, cashew nuts are shelled commercially by very skilled and patient people who have learned the cashew-shelling technique as a trade. In Africa and Brazil, cashews are shelled by machine. The kernel, once removed from its shell, needs further work: after drying it, its reddish-brown outer coating is peeled, either manually or mechanically. The kernels are then graded and vacuum packed for export. Most cashews are dry- or oil-roasted, although raw cashews are available in some specialty stores.

THE USE OF CASHEWS IN AYURVEDIC MEDICINE

Ayurveda is an ancient Indian tradition of medicine that probably originated about 600 B.C. and became known for its many herbal medicines for chronic diseases. Soon after the introduction of cashew nuts to India by the Portuguese in the sixteenth century, cashew nuts became a favorite food and healing agent of Ayurvedic medicine. Cashew nuts are still considered in India to be a good stimulant, an appetizer, a rejuvenator, a hair tonic, an aphrodisiac, and a restorative of lost vigor and sexual health.

Beyond the edible kernel, John Heinerman, in *Heinerman's Encyclopedia of Nuts, Berries and Seeds*, tells us that in Ayurvedic medicine, various parts of the cashew nuts were used as an antidote against poisonous snakebites. He further tells us that in Nigeria, the nut-shell liquid is used as a remedy for skin problems and that the Japanese are testing the same oil for possible use to fight dental cavities.

THE NUTRITIONAL PROPERTIES OF CASHEWS

The edible cashew kernel is a well-balanced nut that belongs to the high-monounsaturated-fat group of nuts, together with almonds, hazelnuts, macadamias, pecans, pine nuts, and pistachios. We can expect cashews to have similar health benefits to the ones shown in clinical studies on almonds. This means that cashews are valuable as a part of any diet for healthy hearts and cholesterol control. They are also very high in plant sterols (over 95 milligrams in an ounce). Cashews have a higher percentage of carbohydrate than the other common nuts.

Cashews, like their tropical cousins the Brazil nuts, are among the high gamma-tocopherol nuts (about 1.5 milligrams in an ounce), making them ideal to mix with almonds or hazelnuts, the high alpha-tocopherol nuts. The possible role of cashews in the prevention of colon cancer in Southern India could be due to their content of gamma-tocopherol, but, at this time, this remains to be confirmed. Cashew nuts are also a reasonable source of delta-tocopherol (just over .1 milligram in an ounce). They contain about .05 milligram of beta-tocopherol and just a trace amount of alpha-tocopherol.

Cashew nuts, which, like Brazil nuts, grow in tropical terrain, contain more selenium than European or North-American nuts—usually about 30 micrograms. Just like with Brazil nuts, their selenium content depends on the soil in which they are grown. Cashews contain about 4.5 grams of protein per ounce. They are very high in the amino acid arginine, containing about 500 milligrams per ounce. One ounce of cashews contains about 1 gram of fiber. An ounce of cashews also contains about 20 micrograms of folic acid, about 14 milligrams of calcium, and about 160 milligrams of potassium.

9

Hazelnuts— The Cool Woodlands Nuts

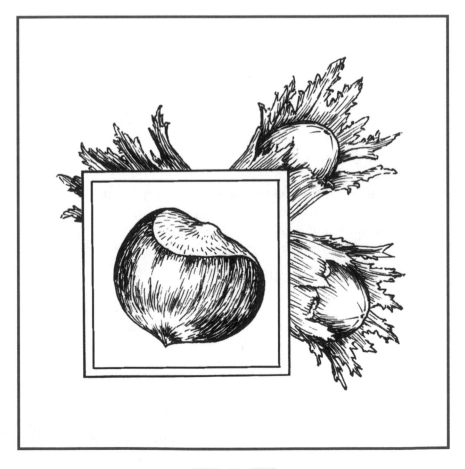

Hazelnuts and their close relatives are part of the wild flora of many regions of Europe, Asia, Africa, and the Americas. Hazelnuts grow on shrubs that grow well in cool, deciduous woodlands, as they love cool, somewhat moist weather, even though in Turkey they grow on rocky hillsides. The variety that grows wild in Europe, particularly in the Mediterranean region and in the Balkans, is the *Corylus avellana* or *Corylus maxima*, while in North America we find the American hazel (*Corylus americana*) and the beaked hazel (*Corylus rostrata*). Hazelnuts are often called filberts as they ripen in August around St. Philibert Day. Another name for hazelnuts, not used too often today, is *cob nuts*.

At times, we find hazelnut trees that grow to a fair size, like the Turkish Tree Hazel, that can grow to a height of 120 feet. All the many species of hazelnut shrubs and trees—at least fifteen of them around the world—produce edible nuts, but some of them produce a much smaller nut than the typical hazelnut on the market today.

The hazelnut has a husk around the shell that is very unusual and quite different from most other tree nuts; it is almost like a beautifully designed sheet of paper that packages the nut. Edwin Menninger in his *Edible Nuts of the World* tells us that "In days gone by the nut was called a *filbert* if the husk was longer than the nut, a *cob* if nut and husk were much the same length, and *hazel* if the husk was very short."

Hazelnut shrubs in the woods of many regions of the earth are a favorite staple of squirrels and other animals, a reminder of the tremendous storehouse of nutritional power in a nutshell.

HAZELNUTS IN HISTORY

Throughout history, hazelnuts have been considered a symbol of wisdom and knowledge. According to Mary Reed, author of *Fruits and Nuts in Symbolism and Celebration*, in Celtic myth, the hazel symbolized inspiration and magical powers.

Hazelnuts, together with other fruits, were gathered in the woods of prehistoric Britain. Timothy Darvill, in his book *Prehistoric Britain*, tells us that during excavations in the Somerset Levels, a vessel still full of hazelnuts was found smashed, probably dropped by the gatherers who were then unable to take the hazelnuts back with them to some distant site.

Hazelnuts have a rich lore, and many myths surround them. References to them abound in ancient Greek and Roman writings and mythology and in the Bible, where they are mentioned for their nutritional and healing power. Pliny, who wrote about plants in the first century after Christ, and Theophrastus, a Greek philosopher probably born in 371 B.C., who was a leader of the Peripatetics and a teacher of botany and natural history, both wrote about hazelnuts.

Much later in the Spain of the seventeenth century, after chocolate was brought in from the New World, the preparation of a pot of chocolate included adding hazelnuts and almonds. This link of hazelnuts to chocolate and pastry is very much alive today: Hazelnuts are used in many chocolate products and are a top choice of many pastry chefs when preparing desserts that contain chocolate.

Lucy Gerspacher, in her book *Hazelnuts and More,* tells us that according to a manuscript found in China from the year 2838 B.C., hazelnuts were considered one of China's five sacred foods. Hazelnuts, like almonds, were used to make milk in ancient China.

John Heinerman, in *Heinerman's Encyclopedia of Nuts, Berries, and Seeds,* tells us that in North America, hazelnuts and some of its botanical relatives were consumed by natives of the lower Illinois River Valley as far back as 6400 B.C. Archeologists found proof of this at a site in Illinois where many archeological treasures have been discovered called the Koster site. Much later, in the 1600s, the Native Americans of Virginia prepared what they considered to be a very healthy nut milk made from hazelnuts. Just as the Europeans of that period used almonds, pine nuts, and walnuts, the American Indians added this hazelnut milk to dishes prepared with the meat of wild deer or to sweet potatoes and other vegetables, a way to make their dishes healthier.

It was between 1858 and 1885 that hazelnuts were planted in Oregon. They later developed into a major crop for this state, which is known for its many wonderful fruits. The hazelnut is now Oregon's official nut. The first tree was planted in 1858 in the Umpqua Valley by British sailor Sam Strictland. Then trees were grown in the Willamette Valley from seeds brought from France by Frenchman David Gernot. But it was not until 1885 that another French farmer, Felix Gillet, brought to Oregon the variety of hazelnuts that are now extensively grown in the state that produces most of the hazelnuts sold in the United States today.

CULTIVATING THE HAZELNUT

The two major hazelnut-growing areas are Turkey and Oregon of the United States. The difference between the way the two regions harvest hazelnuts is intriguing. In Turkey, the largest hazelnut producer in the world, hazelnuts are planted in an uneven fashion on rocky, steep hillsides in clumps of four or five bushes. There are no typical "orchards," in contrast with Oregon, where the orchards are carefully designed. In Turkey, the agricultural techniques are primitive, and the nuts are hand-harvested before they drop to the ground. In the Pacific Northwest, hazelnut farming is done by machine: the nuts are mechanically harvested off the ground.

At one time in Oregon, wild bushes of hazelnuts grew along fence rows and fascinated young children with their tiny edible nuts, which were much smaller than the ones grown commercially today.

THE NUTRITIONAL PROPERTIES OF HAZELNUTS

Hazelnuts are among the nuts high in monounsaturated fat, and we can expect from them the health benefits of other high mono nuts. Hazelnuts are quite similar in composition to almonds and are high in alpha-tocopherols (over 7.5 milligrams in an ounce) and contain a reasonable amount of beta-tocopherol (over .2 milligram in an ounce). An ounce of hazelnuts contains just over a milligram of gamma-tocopherol and .05 milligram of delta-tocopherol. Hazelnuts contain about 4 grams of protein and 2.5 grams of fiber per ounce. One ounce of hazelnuts also contains about 25 micrograms of folic acid, about 30 milligrams of plant sterols, about 55 milligrams of calcium, and about 200 milligrams of potassium.

10

Macadamia Nuts— From Australia to Hawaii

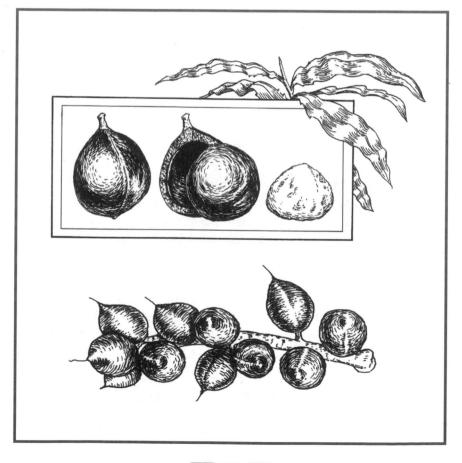

A favorite food of the Australian aborigines, the macadamia nut (*Macadamia integrifolia* and related species) is a native of the subtropical rain forests of Queensland and New South Wales of Australia. It has been called the "Queensland nut" and the "Australian nut." Although the macadamia nut was discovered and named by botanists in the mid-1800s, it was not until the 1950s, over a century later, that Australian farmers began to consider this nut an important crop.

Explorer Friedrich Leichhars, who came to Australia from Prussia, led expeditions to Queensland and discovered macadamia nuts. Another German, Baron Ferdinand Jakob Heinrich Von Mueller, moved to Australia in 1847 after completing his doctorate at the University of Kiel in Germany and named this nut in honor of his friend Dr. John Macadam. Advised to move to warmer climates because of his health, Von Mueller collected and named many native plants unknown in Europe. He became very famous, and rivers and mountains in Australia are named after him.

Macadamias were introduced to Hawaii in the 1880s, and you can still find some of the trees that were brought there in those days, a reminder of the long life and vigor of the macadamia tree. When William Herbert Purvis from Scotland introduced macadamias to Hawaii, he was only 23 years old and the manager of the Pacific Sugar Mill, which produced cane sugar on the big island of Hawaii.

While Hawaii and Australia remain the major producers of macadamia nuts, they are also grown today in subtropical regions like South Africa and Central America.

Rosemary Stanton, a nutritionist in the Department of Medicine at the University of New South Wales in Sydney, Australia, looks with sadness at the fact that the macadamia is not as popular as it should be in its native land, as health messages about nuts and fats have confused people about the proper nutritional value of nuts. She looks forward to the time when macadamias will regain their proper place in the Australian diet.

THE NUTRITIONAL PROPERTIES OF MACADAMIA NUTS

Have you ever heard of palmitoleic acid? Probably not. Even scientists do not talk much about it in relation to nutrition and health. It is a fatty acid, just like its more widely studied sister, oleic acid— the basic type of fat in many nuts, olives, and avocados. Palmitoleic acid is present in very small amounts in most foods, and macadamia nuts are one of the few foods containing a reasonable amount of it—about 16 percent of the nut is palmitoleic acid, close to 5 grams in an ounce. Palmitoleic acid makes macadamias unique, as no other common nut comes even close to macadamias in content of this compound: all the other common nuts described in this book have from 0.2- to 0.4-percent palmitoleic acid, about forty to eighty times less than the macadamia nut.

It seems as though palmitoleic acid is replacing most of the polyunsaturated fats in this nut, making it the nut with the highest percentage of monounsaturated fat. More clinical studies need to be done to understand the role in health of this unique type of fat. We have seen that preliminary studies show that macadamia nuts do lower blood cholesterol, (see page 48), so palmitoleic acid must be a friendly fat.

Macadamia nuts contain about 3 grams of protein for every ounce of nuts. One ounce of macadamia nuts also contains about 3 grams of fiber and 5 micrograms of folic acid. There are also about 20 milligrams of calcium and 100 milligrams of potassium in an ounce of macadamia nuts.

11

Pecans—
The North American
Nuts

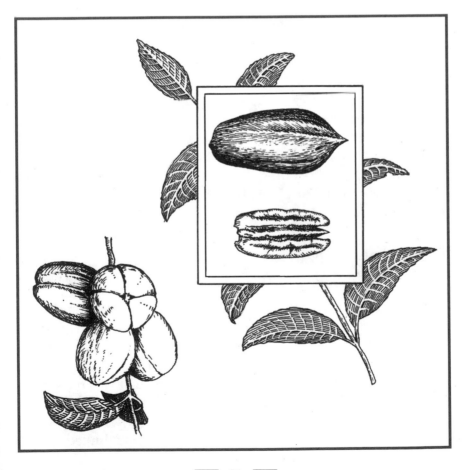

T he pecan, *Carya illinoinensis*, is part of the large *Juglandaceae* family, as is the walnut, as you will see in Chapter 14. Pecan trees are indigenous to a much wider area of North America than the southern regions of the United States we usually associate with this nut. Historians are not certain whether the pecan originated in the northern part of the United States and then slowly expanded to the more southern regions where most of the pecans are grown now, or pecans were native to a wider area of North America from the very beginning.

A STAPLE OF NATIVE AMERICANS

The history of pecans is closely related to the history of Native Americans. In the southern central United States, pecans were a staple of Native Americans since ancient times. American Indians knew, as did many ancient people, that they could collect this precious nut, full of what today we would call "nutritional goodness," and keep it for long periods in its shell—a shell that seals in the goodness, prevents spoilage, and seals out damaging pests and oxygen. Pecans were carefully stored to be used when there was a shortage of other foods. Jasper Woodroof in his book, *Tree Nuts,* tells us that the American Indians traded pecans for other goods and that, as they traveled, they planted pecan trees near their campsites to provide trading capital for their descendants. Careful selection was made for plants that would yield the largest pecans with a thin shell.

PECANS IN THE 1800s

While the Native Americans' planting of pecans near their campsites could be considered the beginning of pecan farming in the United States, most of the pecans early Native Americans and early European settlers ate were from wild trees. Even though George Washington planted pecans, which he called "Mississippi nuts," in the late 1700s, as did Thomas Jefferson, it was only in the late nineteenth century that pecans became cultivated on a large scale.

While some pecan trees were grafted (a bud linked with a

growing plant) in the early 1800s, it was a slave, Antoine, a gardener in Louisiana, whose grafting in 1846 or 1847 of pecan scions (twigs containing buds used in grafting) to young pecan plant stock resulted in major improvement in the quality of the wild nut and the productivity of the tree. This method was forgotten until the art of grafting pecans was revived in 1877, when grafted stock and seedlings (pecan trees grown from seeds) made possible the successful growth of pecan farming. Today, pecans are grown in many countries from Australia to Canada, India, Israel, West Africa, and Mexico.

FROM PECAN MILKS TO PECAN PIES

Nut milks made from pecans were used by the North American Indians, just like almond, hazelnut, pine nut, walnut, and other nut milks were used by the Chinese and Europeans of past centuries. In the days before our modern high-powered kitchen blenders and food processors, pecans were pounded with a mortar and pestle, then water was added and blended well with the finely ground pecans to yield a delicate milk. The Native Americans knew the value of these nut milks that we have encountered in Europe and China over the ages, a reminder that nut milk needs to become a much more important part of the modern diet. These nut milks were easy to digest for the very young, sick, and aging, and provided lasting energy for everyone.

In more recent history, since the Europeans settled in the southern regions of the United States, pecans have been a key food for years in bakery products from fruitcakes to pies. The pecan pie is the best known example of these baked products.

THE NUTRITIONAL PROPERTIES OF PECANS

The pecan is high in gamma-tocopherol (about 8 milligrams in an ounce) and monounsaturated fats. Its high gamma-tocopherol content makes it a good nut to combine with almonds and hazelnuts—the alpha-tocopherol nuts. Pecans contain about 2 grams of protein and just over 2 grams of fiber per ounce. An ounce of pecans also contains 10 micrograms of folic acid, about 1 microgram of alpha-tocopherol, and traces of beta- and delta-tocopherols. Pecans are moderate in plant sterols (over 40 milligrams in an ounce), calcium (10 milligrams in an ounce), and potassium (about 110 milligrams in an ounce).

12

Pine Nuts—
The Aromatic Nuts

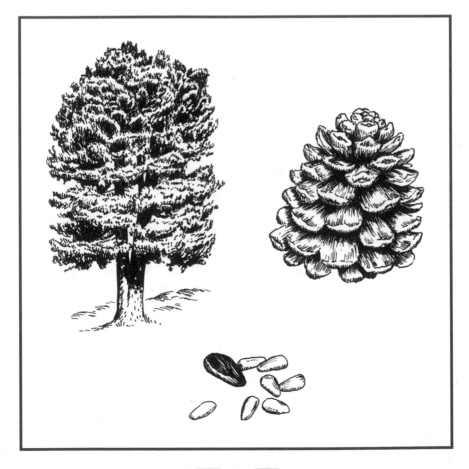

Pine nuts are found everywhere in the world where pine trees grow. There are about eighty different pine trees in the northern hemisphere, and they are found over a wide range of latitudes, from cool northern climates to more temperate regions. As there are so many types of pines, the composition of pine nuts varies somewhat according to the kind of pine tree that bears them and the region in which they grow.

Pine nuts were an important food of the Anasazi Indians of the mountainous regions of New Mexico and Colorado. Also, Dr. John Heinerman tells us in his book *Heinerman's Encyclopedia of Nuts, Berries, and Seeds* that when visiting the Hopi Indian Reservation in Northwest Arizona, he saw a tea being made from pine nuts by a Hopi Indian woman for her clan in 1981.

In Europe the better known nut is from the Italian stone pine (*Pinus pinea*), known in cooking under various names, including pignoli, pignolias, or pinoni. This is the most common type of pine nut on the market. In Australia, we find an unusual pine nut, the bunya nut from the bunya-bunya pine (*Araucaria bidwilli*). In the United States and Mexico, pine nuts are often called *piñon* or *pinyon*. In the Southwest of the United States, the seed of the Colorado pynion (*Pinus edulis*) was a key nut for those populations, together with other pine nuts from different pine trees, like the single leaf pynion (*Pinus monophylla*).

You may find, as the squirrels do, pine nuts on digger pines (*Pinus sabiniana*) on the Eastern slopes of the Sierra Nevada in California, on sugar pines (*Pinus lambertiana*) on mountain ranges of the Pacific Coast, and on ponderosa pines (*Pinus ponderosa*) found from British Columbia in Canada to Baja California in Mexico. And these are just a few of the pine-nut-bearing trees. Many of these nuts were a major source of protein and energy for those living in these regions in early times, along with acorns and walnuts.

While all nuts have their own distinctive flavor, the common pine nuts are particularly aromatic and remind us of the delicate aroma of pine trees. That's probably why they have found their place next to spices and kitchen herbs in many dishes. A well-known modern use of pine nuts that originated in Italy and has spread around the world as Mediterranean cooking became more and more popular, is Italian pesto, a classic sauce for pasta made with pine nuts, olive oil, and basil. Because pine nuts are so aromatic, they have been, and are today, very popular in Mediterranean countries as part of meat, fish, and vegetable dishes. They are also widely used today by the confectionery industry, often in preparing delightful chocolates.

PINE NUTS IN ANCIENT COOKING

Gavius Apicius, born in 25 B.C., who was known in Roman times for giving sumptuous banquets, wrote various cookbooks in Latin, such as *De Re Coquinaria Libri Decem* (Ten Books About Cooking). Among his recipes is one for a sauce for a chicken dish. In this recipe, pine nuts, crushed with pepper, are key ingredients.

Roman pastry, which was often based on ancient Greek recipes, included *domestic cakes* in which pine nuts or walnuts were mixed with dates (from North Africa, then a part of the Roman Empire) and cooked spelt (a type of ancient wheat). Other times, pine nuts were combined with honey and raisin wine, a very sweet wine made from fermented raisins. Both dates and raisins were important components of Roman diets.

Reay Tannahill, in the book *Food in History*, tells us that in Imperial Rome, *asafoetida*, the brown, strong-smelling juice of a giant fennel imported from Persia, was used as a flavoring, but was quite expensive. Apicius suggested storing the asafoetida in a jar of pine nuts and then using a few of the pine nuts in cooking in its place.

Because of its high energy and protein content, like other nuts, pine nuts made a great food for the Roman legions at the peak of Roman power. There was no better combination than nuts, breads, and dried fruits such as raisins for an army in ancient times. And the pine nuts were ready to eat. The ancients had found out through trial and error how well the nutrients of the pine nuts balanced a meal with the other staple of Roman armies—whole-grain bread. A great advantage to an army traveling over hundreds of miles in ancient times was that nuts kept well and could be eaten raw. And in ancient China, milk was made from pine nuts, as well as from almonds and hazelnuts.

PINE NUTS IN MEDIEVAL COOKING

Just as we find almonds in recipes brought back to life in *Curye on Inglysch* (see page 64), so do we find pine nuts. One recipe is for a dish of eels. After stripping the eels of their skin and cutting them in thin pieces, they were fried in olive oil together with pine nuts. Sugar and ginger powder were added, along with ground blanched almonds, white wine, cloves, mace (an aromatic spice made from the covering of the kernel of nutmeg), and pepper, and everything was boiled together.

In another recipe from the same book, wine, pears, toasted bread, sugar or raw honey, and fried pine nuts are boiled and seasoned with pepper and salt, then dressed with mace, cloves, and ginger. And in a *pynnonade*, fried pine nuts were combined with blanched almonds and beaten eggs yolks. Sugar rounded out this recipe for what appeared to be a kind of dessert.

THE AUSTRALIAN PINE NUT

Almost unknown to most people today is an unusual pine nut native to Australia, the bunya nut. Typical bunya trees (*Araucaria bidwilli*) have huge cones that often weigh over five pounds. Bunya pines are found today in countries other than Australia and grow well in climates like that of California, where people grow the bunya tree as an ornamental, without realizing that its nuts are edible. Some bunya trees in my garden bear their huge cones every four or five years, and when the cones fall to the ground, the squirrels don't waste any time tearing them apart and taking the nuts to their hiding places. The bunya nut was a staple food for the Australian aborigines.

THE NUTRITIONAL PROPERTIES OF PINE NUTS

The nutritional composition of pine nuts given below is for the European pine nut that is the most commonly used in today's cooking.

The amount of polyunsaturated fats in pine nuts is about twice that of monounsaturated fat, but pine nuts are still a good source of monounsaturated fat. Of the common tree nuts we have visited in this book, pine nuts are the only ones that contain about the same amount of alpha- and gamma-tocopherols—about 4 milligrams of each in an ounce. They contain only traces of beta- and delta-tocopherols. Let's remember that each type of pine tree produces a nut that is somewhat different in composition.

Pine nuts are very high in protein. An ounce contains about 5 grams of protein. An ounce also contains about 1,000 milligrams of the important amino acid arginine. Pine nuts contain about 2 grams of fiber in an ounce. An ounce of pine nuts also contains about 15 micrograms of folic acid, 4 milligrams of calcium, and 250 milligrams of potassium. As there are so many varieties of pine nuts, the values given for their nutrients are average values of pine nuts from different regions.

The Native Americans of the Southwest often used pine nuts for the treatment of diarrhea, and a tea made from pine nuts was used for head colds. These medicinal uses are still utilized today.

13

Pistachios— Nuts Fit for a Queen

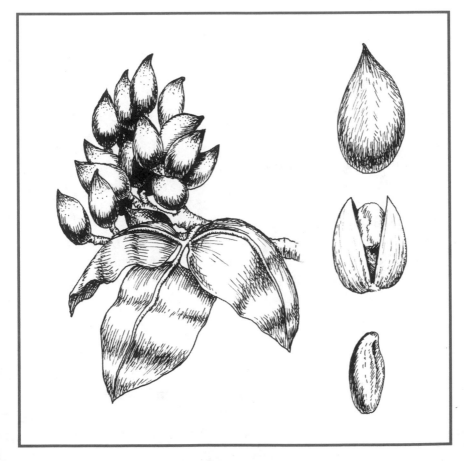

From Persia and surrounding regions—that hub of ancient civilizations where so many of our tree nuts originate— comes the pistachio (*Pistacia vera*). It belongs to the same family as the cashew (*Anacardiaceae*). There are several varieties of pistachios, but only the *Pistachio vera* has a seed that is large enough to be pleasant and acceptable to consumers. Some small-seed varieties of pistachios are eaten locally in some regions but are hardly known anywhere else. Pistachio trees are very hardy and can grow with little rainfall, such as occurs in Middle Eastern deserts and in rocky terrain.

The Queen of Sheba, who lived at the time of King Solomon in the southern part of ancient Arabia, held pistachio nuts in such high esteem that she demanded that all the pistachios produced in her land be given to her and her court, and she hoarded the bulk of the crop for herself. Did she hoard these nuts because they made her and her court healthier and helped them digest their rich meals? It is possible that nuts have such digestive aid properties, but more research is needed to confirm this to be true. Legend has it that lovers met beneath pistachio trees to hear the nuts crack open on moonlit nights for the promise of good fortune.

According to some Roman writers, pistachios probably arrived in Italy and Europe at the time of the birth of Christ and were brought there by the Roman Emperor Vitellius. Other historians believe that pistachios were introduced by the Arabs into Sicily, where today there are extensive plantations. Pistachios probably were taken to China along the ancient Silk Road that linked China to the Mediterranean countries.

It was not until the late 1920s that pistachio seeds were brought to the United States to start what would become a major California nut crop. From the writings of Noel Vietmeyer, a scientist who writes extensively about the history of foods from plants, we learn the story of how the pistachio came to California.

In 1927, alfalfa was dying in the fields of the Midwest and California. A wilt fungus was rotting our primary pasture legume. Farmers were in despair. The situation appeared cata-strophic, and the U.S. Department of Agriculture was besieged with demands to do something. Although there seemed to be no cure, there was one ray of hope. Several years earlier Nikolai Vavilov, the great Russian geneticist, had gathered wild alfalfa in its native habitat in Central Asia; a few of his collected strains showed slight wilt resistance. He offered to help American agronomists collect more alfalfa from the Asian site, and the USDA staff in Washington was more than willing to send plant explorers. But they were thwarted because the U.S. had no diplomatic relations with the 10-year old Soviet government.

An alfalfa expert, Harvey Westover, was sent to the then Soviet Union to work with a Russian botanist and bring back varieties of alfalfa that are known to be resistant to the disease that plagued the American crops. William Whitehouse, a 36-year-old New Englander, botanist and an expert in fruit trees, was sent along to search for fruit crops. It was known that many of our common fruits originated in Russia, Persia and the surrounding regions. Persia was known for its many varieties of pistachios and Whitehouse could learn how they were grown and handled and hopefully bring back some seeds of the better varieties.

Whitehouse and Westover were told that their mission was unofficial, and the State Department could not help them should something happen to them. Thanks to Vavilov, they succeeded in finding alfalfa seeds that would resist the wild fungus that was destroying the American crops, and with this major goal accomplished, Whitehouse can now sneak into Persia alone in the quest for the best pistachio seeds. In the ancient suqs [North African marketplaces] of Teheran, Isfahan, and Kerman, and in dusty village markets, he sifts through the piles of produce. For almost six months the lone scientist wandered in this land of sand and dust and dirt. He was told to. . .make his clothes blend with those of the Persians. Water was often a luxury, bathrooms were nonexistent, the food was often suspect. He toured pistachio plantations and pored through suqs looking at all the pistachios he could find. One day, near the city of Rafsanjan, his fingers closed over a particular nut. It is big. It is round. The shell is nicely split at one end. He drops it into his collecting bag.

Eventually his botanic booty amounted to about 20 pounds of individually selected seed, and in 1930 he carried them out of Persia and back to Washington. Within a year he had germinated them and was growing them under observation at the USDA Plant Introduction Station at Chico, California. However, pistachio trees take 7 to 10 years to mature, so it was almost a decade before Whitehouse could get much idea of what he had gathered. Out of the 3,000 trees grown from the seeds he collected, only 20 were worth keeping, only 3 were promising enough to name, and 2 of those subsequently proved unsatisfactory.

Thus, of all the seeds that Whitehouse had collected during six months of hardship, only one proved useful. The sole remaining tree was from that special seed from the city of Rafsanjan. He never saw the tree it came from. He had picked the seed out of a pile of drying nuts in the orchards of the Agah family, prominent pistachio growers at Rafsanjan in Iran's central plateau.

In the 1950s, when the tree was beginning to show exceptional promise, Whitehouse named it "Kerman," for the famous carpet-making city near Rafsanjan. He asked his superiors in Washington to allocate funds for developing it into a commercial crop. They balked, claiming that no money was available for pistachio. Find another project, he was told; pistachio would never become a viable crop in this country. The state of California was even less enthusiastic. As Whitehouse's colleague, Lloyd Joley, [a USDA horticulturist] remembers, "There never was much interest in our work. I myself never expected to see a pistachio industry in my lifetime."

But Whitehouse never lost his enthusiasm or dedication. Although stationed in Maryland, he traveled to California every year for three decades to spend several weeks working with Joley, sharing the tedious work of hand pollination and grafting—doggedly plugging away at pistachio improvement.

Developing a new crop, especially a tree crop, is a monumental achievement, and the pair faced frequent setbacks and frustrations. Each time they planted a seed they had to wait five years before blossoms formed so they could tell even what sex their tree was. Severe disease rotted the roots of their trees, even attacking those of the "Kerman" tree. Some plants grew vigorously and looked marvelous, only to produce few nuts; some failed to ripen their seeds all at the same time; others yielded well initially, only to decline in subsequent years. "We would get good results one year and then couldn't repeat them the next," recalls Joley. "Every time something like that happened the pressures to cancel the program rose. Almost everyone said it would never amount to anything."

Nevertheless, the lone "Kerman" tree continued growing and yielding well. The beleaguered scientists had that alone to keep them going. Only its consistently strong growth, its large, good tasting seeds and high proportion of split shells—very desirable because they make the nuts easy to open—made the seemingly mad, decades-long ordeal worthwhile. Eventually they discovered that related pistachio species resisted root-rot fungi and made good rootstock. Soon they were taking buds from the "Kerman" tree and grafting them onto seedlings of these hardy species. By the late 1950s, some 30 years after the initial collection, a pistachio industry was becoming somewhat feasible; the two pioneers had a good female tree and they had disease-resistant types to use as rootstock. But a third botanical ingredient was missing—a good male tree that would provide pollen at exactly the same time that the female was in flower.

Whitehouse had brought from Iran the seed of a female tree. Almost by accident a grower from the Fresno area discovered a very prolific male tree, prolific with male flowers. It turned out that the timing was almost exactly perfect.

Today pistachios are grown successfully on small and large farms in California, and the United States is the biggest supplier of the delicious nuts to the world.

PISTACHIOS IN MEDIEVAL COOKING

Just like almonds and pine nuts, pistachios were used in recipes of fourteenth-century England in heavy meat dishes. In *Curye on*

Inglysch, we find a pastry dish well filled with various wild meats and birds, combined with dates soaked in honey and plenty of pistachios chopped or coarsely minced. This pistachio recipe reminds us that nuts were key ingredients of meat cooking in medieval England. The chefs knew that nuts made their meat dishes not only more delectable, but also healthier and easier to digest.

Once again, we learn that people in earlier times knew how to combine foods for better health much before our modern knowledge of the chemistry of foods told us about the saturated fats of meats and the unsaturated fats of nuts and seeds.

THE NUTRITIONAL PROPERTIES OF PISTACHIOS

An ounce of pistachios contains 6 grams of protein, 3 grams of fiber, about 15 micrograms of folic acid, .5 milligram of alpha-tocopherol, a whopping 7.5 milligrams of gamma-tocopherol, and traces of beta- and delta-tocopherols. It also contains almost 60 milligrams of plant sterols, 40 milligrams of calcium, and 310 milligrams of potassium.

14

Walnuts— The Royal Nuts

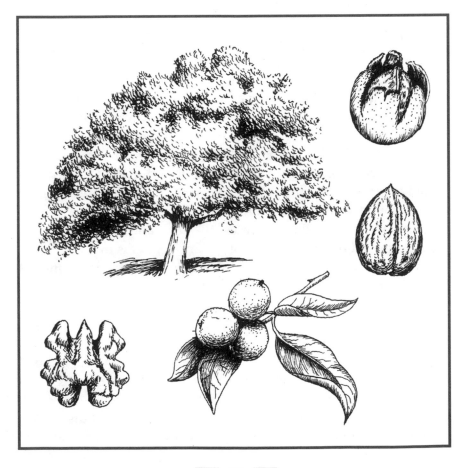

There are different varieties of walnuts in Asia, Europe, and the Americas. They all belong to the same large walnut family, the *Jugandaceae*. The most widely cultivated walnut and best known is the Persian walnut, *Juglans regia*. This is the walnut most commonly known to you and I—the one we call simply, walnut. *Regia*, in Latin, means belonging to royalty. This is a sign of the high esteem in which Persian walnuts were held in ancient Rome. Native to the Americas is the black walnut *Juglans nigra* (*nigra*, meaning black in Latin), an important food of Native Americans in both North and South America. The butternut, *Juglans cinerea*, or American white walnut, almost unknown to many today, was well known to the Narragansett Indians, who used its oil for flavoring and the nuts to thicken their soups or stew of vegetables and sometimes meat. In Japan, we find the Japanese walnut, *Juglans ailanthifolia*. Other nuts are called "walnuts" even though they are not *Juglans*, like the African walnut, *Coula edulis*, found in the Sierra Leone region in Africa.

Walnuts were found in prehistoric deposits in Europe dating back to the Iron Age (which began around the eighth century B.C.). Pliny the Elder who lived between A.D. 23 and 79 and who was a Roman scholar and naturalist and wrote the thirty-seven-volume *Historia Naturalis*, tells us that, from Persia, walnuts had already been introduced into Italy before the birth of Christ. Exceptionally well-preserved unshelled walnuts were found during the excavation of the ruins of Pompei and Ercolano. These cities near Naples in Italy, founded in the sixth or early fifth century B.C., were prosperous resorts with villas, temples, theaters, and spas. Both cities were destroyed by the eruption of Mount Vesuvius in A.D. 79.

And walnuts and their oil were highly prized in ancient Greece, where they were common at least four centuries before Christ.

Much later, British merchant marines transported walnuts to ports around the world with their ships, and the Persian walnut became known as the English walnut. Just like with the almond that originated in the same part of the world, Franciscan fathers brought the walnut to Mexico and later to California. Today, the Central Valley of California is a major producer of walnuts.

Persian walnuts were imported to China during the Han

Dynasty (about 200 B.C. to A.D. 220), a dynasty noted for its support of literature and the arts, and now China is a major producer of walnuts.

WALNUTS—BRAIN, STRENGTH, AND HEALING FOOD?

As the kernel of walnuts resembles in appearance the human brain, walnuts have been considered brain food for centuries. For the same reason, and because of their hard shell, the Greeks called walnuts *caryon* from *kara*, which means head. When the Doctrine of Signatures (a doctrine that taught that the healing or beneficial effects of herbs and plants were related to their resemblance to parts of the body) was widely used in medicine in the sixteenth and seventeenth centuries, walnuts were considered a food for the brain and to boost intellect when eaten.

The walnut-human brain connection is found in other early uses of walnuts. An English herbalist, William Cole, suggested in 1657 to lay upon the crown of the head a bruised kernel of a walnut moistened with wine. John Heinerman in *Heinerman's Encyclopedia of Nuts, Berries, and Seeds*, tells us that when in China, he saw stocky, muscular wrestlers eating walnuts before entering the ring. And walnuts are an integral part of many folk remedies in China.

The leaves and the green hull of the walnut have been used for centuries as folk remedies. One classic folk remedy in Germany for runny noses and sinus problems is a tea made with walnut leaves, which is also used externally as a wash for skin problems. A tea made from walnut leaves is very astringent, and it has been used as a skin lotion and as a gargle in relieving skin irritations, the itching of insect bites, and sore throats.

THE NUTRITIONAL PROPERTIES OF WALNUTS

Walnuts are high in polyunsaturated fats, which are valuable for good health but are also more sensitive to damage by oxygen than monounsaturated fats. In her wisdom, Nature has made the oil of the walnut rich in that great antioxidant, gamma-tocopherol (over 8 milligrams in an ounce), which not only protects the oil from rapid spoilage, but also adds nutritional benefits for us. And walnuts, among all the tree nuts, are the best sources of delta-tocopherol (.65 milligram in an ounce), an antioxidant that is a close sister of vitamin E but in need of more research to determine its healthful benefits. They also contain traces of alpha- and beta-tocopherols.

The polyunsaturated fats of the walnut are rich in omega-3 oils, an important type of polyunsaturated fat. This makes walnuts an excellent source of these fats for vegetarians who do not eat fish, one of the animal sources of omega-3.

"Walnuts," says Dr. Sabaté of Loma Linda University in California, "have a nice percentage of alpha-linolenic acid which is an omega-3, and this is the precursor of EPA [eicosapentaenoic acid] and DHA [docosahexaenoic acid], two fatty acids that are found in fish and fish oil. We wanted to see if the subjects of one of our studies on walnuts had increased levels in the blood of these fats and we found that, in fact, they had higher levels of these fats. You just need to eat two ounces, a handful, of walnuts a day."

An ounce of walnuts contains about 4 grams of protein, about 1.5 grams of fiber, about 20 micrograms of folic acid, 50 milligrams of plant sterols, about 30 milligrams of calcium, and almost 140 milligrams of potassium.

15

Still More Tree Nuts

There are many other nuts in the world. In his book *Edible Nuts of the World*, Dr. Edwin Menninger describes many nuts from all regions of the earth, most of them unknown to most of us. A few of the tree nuts described by Menninger deserve mention, but from a nutritional point of view, these nuts have little or nothing in common with the typical nuts we have just visited. Chestnuts are mostly carbohydrate, as are acorns from oaks. Cola nuts are stimulant nuts due to their high caffeine content, and ginkgo nuts are hardly known outside of China, although ginkgo has become popular for the use of its leaves as an herbal medicine. Many spices are nuts, including nutmeg.

CHESTNUTS

Chestnuts are found in Europe (*Castanea sativa*), especially in Italy, China (*Castanea mollissima*), the United States (*Castanea dentata*), and other parts of the world. But they are perhaps more popular in Europe, where street vendors sell them roasted along the streets of many cities. The Latin poet Virgil mentions chestnuts as a popular food in ancient Italy. Chestnuts are prepared boiled, roasted, and as a confection, prepared with sugar and sold under the French name of *marron glacé*. The American chestnut was considered sweeter than the European varieties, but a fungus has destroyed much of these trees in North America, limiting their availability today.

Chestnuts have been used over the centuries as a source of energy. Dried chestnuts are a high-carbohydrate food, about 22 grams in an ounce with 3 grams of fiber, and very low in fat, about 1.5 grams. They have about 1.3 grams of protein. If you want a diet based on nuts, combine one of the high-protein tree nuts with high-carbohydrate nuts for a great meal.

ACORNS

It is said that there are 450 kinds of acorns, the nuts of the oak tree. The acorns eaten by Natives Americans include the *Quercus agrifolia, Quercus alba, Quercus virginiana,* and *Quercus lobata* (*Quercus* is Latin for oak). Acorns, like chestnuts, are high-carbohydrate, low-fat, and low-protein nuts. They contain a bitter substance that should be washed out, as Native Americans did, as the first step in the preparation of acorn dishes. In some mission villages, like Pala in San Diego County in southern California, older American Indians still know how to prepare a mush from acorns. This mush is very similar to the corn mush or polenta of Mediterranean countries.

Just like chestnuts, acorns have long been considered an important source of energy for many Native Americans.

COLA NUTS

Cola nuts (*Cola nitida* or *Cola vera*), sometimes called kola nuts, gave the name to, and supplied the caffeine for, cola drinks many years ago, before by-products of the preparation of decaffeinated coffee supplied a cheaper source of caffeine for many of these products. Cola nuts supply caffeine to millions of people in many regions of Africa where the nuts of the cola trees are chewed as stimulants and were used before demanding physical tasks to ensure lasting endurance. It's interesting that today we find decaffeinated cola drinks, a strange name for beverages that took their name from a caffeine nut!

GINKGO NUTS

Ginkgo (*Ginkgo biloba*) is one of the most ancient trees—millions of years old—alive today. It is a native of ancient China, but today, ginkgo trees are grown as ornamental trees in North America, while ginkgo leaves, rather than the nut, are a popular medicinal herb in China, Europe, and the United States. The roasted kernels of the ginkgo nut are highly prized in China. Ginkgo nuts are excellent sources of potassium and niacin and good sources of copper and magnesium.

NUTMEG

Nutmeg (*Myristica fragrans*) is a popular spice, familiar to just about everyone. Sophisticated cooks buy whole nutmegs and grate them with a small grater, similar to a cheese grater, just before using them. It is said that nations have gone to war over this nut. Abundant in the Polynesian islands that are scattered between New Zealand and Hawaii in the central and southern Pacific Ocean, nutmeg has been fought over amongst the Arabs, Portuguese, and the Dutch in past centuries. The natives of some of these islands lost their independence and became almost slaves that cared for the nutmeg plantations. Now nutmeg is also grown in other regions with a similar climate. It probably became popular as a spice as people found it helped digestion and decreased flatulence.

The time has now come to learn how to make nuts part of a healthy diet. In Part Three, we will look at the other foods needed to create a balanced diet, and you will learn some of the many possible ways to make nuts part of a healthy diet.

PART THREE

Tree Nuts in Our Diets

16

The Role of Nuts in a Healthy Diet

In Parts One and Two of this book, we've seen that, over the centuries, nuts had many diverse uses, from snacks straight from the shell to dishes for royalty in Europe to nut milks for infants in China. Since the ancient Chinese considered food to be, as Reay Tannahill points out, ". . . intimately bound up not only with the health of the body, but also with that of the mind and soul," the fact that nuts were held in high esteem takes on even greater significance.

In the Bible, nuts were often mentioned as "some of the best products of the land." Genesis 43:11 says, "Then their father Israel said to them, 'If it must be, then do this: Put some of the best products of the land in your bags and take them down to the man as a gift—a little balm and a little honey, some spices and myrrh, some pistachio nuts and almonds.'" Walnuts were considered healing foods in the Middle Ages, and ancient Greeks considered them to be brain food. Hazelnuts, like walnuts, were considered in Greek and Roman mythology and in the Bible as healing foods.

We have found that Native Americans considered pine nuts and pecans essential components of their diets, Australian aborigines enjoy macadamia nuts as staples in their diets, and cashews are held in high esteem in India. There is no doubt that from ancient times to today, nuts have been part of the human diet.

But things are changing. Dr. Antonia Trichopoulou, professor at the Athens School of Public Health in Greece and chief of the World Health Organization Collaborating Center for Nutrition and Greece National Center for Nutrition, gives us a sad example of these changes in the 1990s using the Greek diet as an example:

> *When I was a child, in the days when Greek men were the oldest living men in the world, I used to put in my pockets almonds, chestnuts, hazelnuts, and dried raisins: that was for my 10 o'clock school break. That was considered a healthy snack for a child, and it was. Unfortunately, this is not done now; parents give the children money, and they buy donuts. Today our men are no longer the oldest in the world."*

Have we lost of the art of eating in our fast-moving computer age? Are we unable to find time for a proper meal of real foods? Dr. Wenche Frølich, a well-known Norwegian nutritionist and writer, tells a story of a Norwegian child who, when asked to draw a picture of a fish, drew a square because the only fish he had ever seen was a frozen square fish steak from a package. Shouldn't we be able to find more time for proper meals in an age where computers are making our lives so much easier and efficient? What an incredible contradiction!

Fortunately, nuts can be part of a quick meal, as well as an elaborate dish. We can eat them on the trail while hiking, during a break at the office or from a tennis match or a soccer game, and we can make them part of our meals. But no matter how easy it is to eat a nut, never forget that we need to find more time for proper meals.

We need to do two things: We need to revisit the foundations of healthy diets. I will address that issue in this chapter. And we need to open the door to the many ways nuts can and should be part of such a diet, which we will discuss in the next chapter.

THE TRUE MEANING OF THE TERM DIET

"Diet" has become a term that implies sacrifice or suffering. To most of us, dieting means following restrictions forced upon us by a major illness like diabetes or heart disease, or something we do to lose weight. "Diet" is something we do not want to keep up for too long.

In this book, I use the term diet in its true meaning—the usual food and drink of a person—rather than as something prescribed for medical reasons. The word diet is derived from the Latin word *diaeta*, which meant way of living.

With this definition of diet in mind, there is no doubt that we need to take two key steps. We need to make plant foods the foundation of our diet and to consume a wide variety of plant foods, from all parts of the plant. We also need to be sure that this diet is enjoyable, or no one is going to follow it for very long. There are easy techniques you can use to be sure that, as you move to a plant-based diet, you do it right. An unbalanced plant-based diet can fail just like a high-animal-food diet.

THE GOODNESS OF PLANT FOODS

Just about every health professional today agrees that a healthy diet is a primarily plant-based diet. They may disagree about how much fat you should eat, or whether or not this diet should be *strictly* vegetarian. But the concept that we need to increase the amount of plant foods in our diets for disease prevention is just about universally accepted.

Dr. Jeffrey Blumberg, professor in the School of Nutrition Science and Policy at Tufts University in Boston, and associate director and chief of the Antioxidants Research Laboratory of the Jean Mayer USDA Human Nutrition Research Center on Aging at Tufts, reminds us that there is no doubt about the value of plant-based diets.

> *I don't think there is any doubt that there is a broad consensus that diets that are largely plant-based, that is, are rich in fruits and vegetables and other plant foods, are associated with better long-term health outcomes, lower risk for several chronic diseases, for example, and even with maintenance of healthy body weights. I really don't think it matters whether you talk about a Mediterranean diet or an Asian diet or a vegetarian diet. They really overlap tremendously when we look at micronutri-*

*ent profiles [such as of vitamins and minerals] or at macronu-
trient profiles, like the fats, and it's clear that the diets that are
lower in saturated fats, yet still generous in the monos and
some of the polys, are repeatedly associated with lower disease
incidence.*

And Dr. Gabriele Riccardi, professor of Metabolic Diseases and
chairman of Applied Dietetics of the School of Medicine at the
University of Naples, Italy—in the heart of the good Mediterranean diet region—reminds us that:

*The Mediterranean diet, a plant-based diet, is associated with
a very high life expectancy and very low incidence of the major
killer diseases of the Western world, like cardiovascular disease
and cancer. The main feature of this diet, at least as it is prac-
ticed in Italy, is a very low content of animal fat and, in general, of animal-derived products. In Italy, the traditional diet
consists of about half the amount of meat as the diet in the
United States and other northern European countries. . . . This
means not just a low-animal-fat diet, but a low-animal-protein
diet as well.*

*Unfortunately, what we are presently observing is that this
diet is changing and, unfortunately, it is changing in the wrong
direction. People do not like to spend too much time cooking, so
they prefer to get fast food, food already prepared that they just
put in the microwave oven and eat. These habits are changing
the traditional way of eating, and the amount of saturated fat is
increasing, the amount of total fat is increasing, and the consumption of legumes, vegetables, and fruit is decreasing in
Italy. This is not a favorable event for our health because what
we expect is that, in parallel, we will also observe an increase in
the cardiovascular disease incidents and all other diseases that
are so prevalent in other affluent societies. We hope [with a
campaign now in progress] to underline the importance of
going back to rediscover our Mediterranean diet tradition.*

Dr. Joan Sabaté, of Loma Linda University emphasizes the
importance of a plant- and nut-based diet:

A plant-based diet is probably the best, and nuts are an essential component of such a diet. Not only are they of plant origin, but they are a group of foods that need to be consumed regularly. Nuts, together with whole grains, legumes [beans, peas, and lentils], fruits, and vegetables, constitute a diet that provides almost every nutrient that we know is necessary, except for vitamin B_{12}, and nuts provide many phytochemicals and other yet-to-be-discovered nutrients that we know are in plant foods.

Dr. Colin Campbell from Cornell University suggests a good and simple system to choose and combine plant foods for the ultimate diet.

The diet should consist of a variety of good-quality, plant-based foods. A simple way to a balanced diet is to choose some foods from each part of the plant: the roots, stems, leaves, seeds, fruits, and even flowers. In other words, I think we should eat all parts of the plant and a variety of different kinds of plants.

In different terms, Dr. David Jenkins, professor of Medicine and Nutritional Sciences at the University of Toronto in Canada, and director of the Risk Factor Modification Center at St. Michael's Hospital in Toronto, where he also serves as a staff physician in the Division of Endocrinology and Metabolism, brings us the same message by suggesting we combine green leaves, root vegetables, fruits, and other seeds, like whole grains and beans, with nuts of all kinds for what he likes to call an *eating program*—a good way to avoid the term "diet."

Now, go a step further to add variety and to ensure a broad intake of nutrients and phytochemicals. Choose more than one type of seed or fruit or leaf or root or stem, and even an occasional edible flower, and be sure that, by the end of the day, you have consumed foods from each part of the plants. It does not matter if you make these combinations part of a single meal, like dinner, or if you have seeds and dried fruits at one meal, like the classic nuts-and-sun-dried-raisins snack; a large green salad and a whole-grain bread sandwich for lunch; a fresh fruit in mid-afternoon, perhaps with a few nuts so you won't be starving by dinnertime; and for dinner, some cooked root vegetables and green leaves (like kale with their stems), broccoli, and fish (or tofu) with a bowl of nuts on the table and a dessert of fresh fruits in season.

GUIDELINES FOR FOLLOWING A NUTRITIOUS PLANT-BASED DIET

Don't fret about changing your way of eating. Following a healthful, plant-based diet can be easy—and delicious! Here are some guidelines to help you follow such a diet.

The Quick Guides—The Food Pyramids

Another way to choose your foods is to use one of the many food guide pyramids. Food pyramids had their birth in Scandinavian countries and have been used in recent years to help people choose their food wisely. There are several to choose from—the United States Department of Agriculture's Food Guide Pyramid, my own Superpyramid, which I developed with nutritionist Dr. Wenche Frølich of Norway and published some years ago, the Traditional Healthy Mediterranean Diet Pyramid developed by the Boston-based Oldways Preservation and Exchange Trust in collaboration with many scientists, and other pyramids developed by various organizations. All teach the same concept—that plant foods should be the foundation of a good meal—and while they differ in some ways, they all emphasize plant foods as the foundation of a healthy diet.

To make things even easier, together with Dr. John Farquhar of Stanford, I created an upside-down pyramid that clearly distinguishes between plant foods and animal foods. (See Figure 16.1 on page 113.)

This figure depicts the Upside-Down Pyramid, with the larger tier—with the foods to be consumed freely as the foundation of the meal—at the top, rather than at the bottom, of the pyramid. This overcomes some people's objections to the concept that the foods to be consumed the *least* are at the *top* of the usual food pyramids— the top tier should be the ultimate location for the *most* desirable

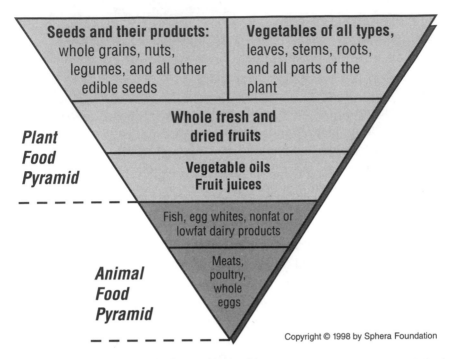

Figure 16.1. The Upside-Down Pyramid. *(Courtesy of the Sphera Foundation.)*

foods. Make some photocopies of this pyramid; put one in your kitchen and take another with you when you travel.

Don't Make Meat, Poultry, or Fish the Center of Your Plate

Meat, poultry, and fish should not be the centerpiece of your plate. Make your whole grains, legumes, fruits, vegetables, and nuts the main portion of your meal, and if you must have meat, poultry, or fish, make these a small side dish. Among these three choices, fish should be your first choice. Fatty fishes like salmon, trout, and swordfish contain beneficial polyunsaturated oils. These oils help to lower blood triglycerides. Fatty fishes are high in omega-3 fats. If weight is a problem, choose low-fat fishes like sole, snapper, and halibut. Shellfish, like shrimp and crab, contain cholesterol, but are very low in fat.

Chicken, beef, pork, lamb, and other meats contain cholesterol and saturated fat. If you do eat them, choose the leanest cuts.

Remember that, per ounce, chicken, with or without skin, contains about as much cholesterol and saturated fat as red meat.

Keep Refined Foods to a Minimum

No nutritionist will disagree with the statement that refined-flour products, like white bread, should not be staples of the diet. But when plant foods become the foundation of the diet, it's more crucial than ever that refined-flour products and other refined grains be minimized in, or eliminated from, the diet. A whole grain is a storehouse of fiber, essential oils, vitamins, minerals, good proteins, and many precious phytochemicals. But to make whole grains acceptable, we need to prepare them properly, an art many of us have lost. Properly flavored with rosemary, sage, and other herbs of your choice, whole-grain pasta and rice taste much better than their refined counterparts. Whole-grain breads free of hydrogenated fats are delicious. Or you can bake your own whole-grain breads at home. For ways to prepare homemade breads with special appeal, read my *Nutrition Secrets of the Ancients*.

Drink Fruit and Vegetable Juices

Go ahead and drink your fruit and vegetable juices; they have a lot of nutritional goodness. But eat plenty of whole vegetables and fruits as well. Just as important, make sure you get most of your sugars from such dried fruits as raisins, figs, dates, and prunes, or from natural, unrefined products like unfiltered, raw honey or unrefined sugar and maple syrup, rather than from fiber-free candies.

Utilize the Power of Herbs and Spices

In all regions of the earth, kitchen herbs from rosemary to ginger and garlic have been used to flavor foods. Until recently, we knew only that they helped us to enjoy our food and make it more flavorful. The flavor of such herbs as sage and rosemary became associated with Mediterranean cuisine, ginger with Indian cooking, and chili pepper with Middle Eastern cooking.

Today we know that in addition to being flavorful, all these herbs and spices contain powerful antioxidants, which are natural food preservatives, and in the days before modern refrigeration, they helped preserve foods in hot climates like India. And we know now that other herbs like garlic contain powerful compounds that have antibiotic properties, that help control blood coagulation, and that help control blood cholesterol when eaten in conjunction with a proper diet. But many of the antioxidants and other compounds in these herbs and spices are also powerful protective factors for heart disease and some types of cancers. Without knowing it, for centuries, people were adding protective factors for their heart and even for cancer prevention.

Use herbs, spices, and garlic freely and regularly to add pleasant protection to your meals.

Bring Back Meal Rituals

For centuries, people, rich or poor, used to take time to eat in a quiet environment. Dinner was the time for a family to get together, to relax, and perhaps to say a prayer.

In the modern world full of rushing and stress, the time for a peaceful dinner, prepared with love, has shrunk and in many cases disappeared. A quickly defrosted, microwave-heated, precooked dinner eaten in hurry is not uncommon in our modern society. What should be reserved for an occasional meal in a special situation has often become a daily routine, just as a fast-food lunch has become the rule, rather than the exception, for many. There is a place for all of this. Find time, at least a few times a week, at the end of a busy day for a peaceful meal full of plant-based dishes!

TREE NUT ALLERGIES

About 99 percent of the American population can eat tree nuts with no problem. According to the Food Allergy Network, less than 1 percent may have some kind of true food allergy to peanuts, and less than 1 percent may have a true allergy to tree nuts. Peanuts are not tree nuts; they are part of the bean family. Some people may be allergic to tree nuts or to one specific tree nut, just as some people are allergic to wheat products. If you think you may be allergic to tree nuts or to any other food, you should consult a health-care professional, as severe allergic reactions to food could cause serious, even life-threatening, medical problems. If you know you have an allergy to nuts, avoid eating them. Read food labels carefully, as nuts and nut products are often used in prepared foods. Sometimes the term allergy is misused, and a negative reaction to a food may actually be an intolerance, where one simply does not have enough of a necessary enzyme to digest that food properly.

NUTS AND OBESITY

In some cases of overweight, dietary restrictions are necessary. In such cases, consult with a health-care professional about the consumption of any food, including nuts. Adding any food to your diet that increases your caloric intake—no matter what the food—may cause weight gain if excessive calorie consumption continues. Nuts should replace other less healthful foods in your diet, and because eating nuts makes you feel satisfied, you'll soon discover that you'll want to eat less of other foods.

LOOKING BEYOND FOOD FOR BETTER HEALTH

Total health is impossible to achieve with food alone. You must also take into account the key roles that physical activity and stress play in good health.

Physical Activity

No matter how great the diet is, the human body was never meant to sit around all day. Physical activity of some kind is a daily need. Since World War II, we have developed more and more ways to cut down our physical efforts, from using a car for almost any outing, to doing our laundry in the washing machine and mowing our lawn with a gas-powered mower. For optimal health, some intense physical activity is imperative on a regular basis—*at least* three or four times a week. From sports like tennis, to jogging, walking, hiking, bicycling, and swimming, to working out at a gym or in an aerobics class, you have literally hundreds of choices to please you.

Stress Relief

Just as important in our modern, fast-moving lives, we must find relief from stress. Again, you can choose from many methods to do so, from organized activities like yoga and other Asian arts to massage, from sitting peacefully reading a book in a quiet room to performing some simple deep breathing exercises. Don't ever say: "I don't have time," because you may have to take much more time off because of a major illness.

You are now ready to find ways to make tree nuts part of a pleasant and healthy diet. Read Chapter 17 for reminders of simple ways of adding them to your meals. Some of them, you might already know. You may also discover ways you never thought of.

17

Endless Uses for Nuts

I t's amazing how few people consider nuts a food that should be a key ingredient in the kitchen and that can be part of an endless number of recipes, from breakfast to dinner. This chapter will give suggestions for a wide variety of ways to use nuts, some very simple, needing practically no preparation, some needing simple cooking for the cook in a hurry, and others for the sophisticated cook or chef with time to cook.

Add nuts to your favorite recipes, create your own recipes, find a good nut recipe in your regular cookbook, or look for nut recipes in some of the books listed in the References section beginning on page 135. Nut councils (see the Sources of Further Information section) will be glad to send you free booklets containing many interesting recipes using their nuts.

A BOWL OF NUTS ON THE DINING TABLE

Placing a bowl of nuts on the dining table is one of the easiest ways to make nuts a part of the diet. In Egypt and the Middle East, this is a favorite way to serve nuts. It's simple and effortless. You may use raw or roasted nuts. If you enjoy cracking nuts, place them on the table in their shells with a nutcracker nearby; otherwise, buy them already shelled. Use a mixture of nuts or simply serve your favorite variety of nuts.

NUTS FOR BREAKFAST

It is easy to add nuts to breakfast meals, as many prepackaged breakfast cereals include nuts as ingredients. In some stores, you may find granola-type cereals. The Swiss have a famous mixture of cereal flakes, nuts, raisins, and dried apples that they call *muesli*; you can make your own, or you can find it premixed. Be sure you purchase whole-grain cereals. Chopped or ground nuts, easy to prepare in a food processor or blender, add both nutrition and flavor to home-cooked cereals like oatmeal. Add dried fruit, like raisins, and something fresh, like bananas, to make your breakfast complete.

If you want to go a step further to make your breakfast cereal a supercereal, serve it with one of the nut milks now available on the market, or make your own. You'll be surprised at the variety of flavors nut milks can add to your breakfast: you could use a different tree nut milk each day!

If you like breakfast meats, try replacing some of them with some nuts. This way, you'll add high-arginine protein to your diet, and replace some of the saturated fats with unsaturated fats.

And, as we have already seen, as with any other meal, a bowl of nuts on the breakfast table goes well with almost any breakfast choice. Nuts alone are also good for breakfast when you are in a hurry.

NUTS AT LUNCH

For lunch, add nuts to your salads and pasta dishes. If you are eating out, choose a nut burger or sandwich made with a slice of nut loaf, or try making one at home. If in a hurry, eat some nuts, bread, and dried or fresh fruit.

NUTS AT DINNER

For a great dinner, start with a salad of dark green lettuce and other leaves and some tomatoes, dressed with a good nut oil or olive oil and vinegar (salt optional). Follow this with a bowl of brown rice or whole-grain pasta and a small portion of fish (or tofu, tempeh, or beans for a vegetarian diet), cooked carrots and broccoli or other root and stem vegetable, and some fresh fruit for dessert. You may add some yogurt or cheese, or replace the fish with some meat or chicken.

LEARNING TO REPLACE SOME ANIMAL PRODUCTS WITH NUTS

One simple thing you can do to improve your diet is to replace some high-fat animal products with nuts in recipes. Do this for every meal or as a first step if you or someone in your house loves high-fat meats, like those used in those typical old-fashioned breakfasts.

Take John for instance. John loved sausage or bacon and eggs for breakfast every morning. His blood cholesterol was high. He was told to cut down on animal fats, but when he cut out the sausage and bacon he was quite dissatisfied. John did not want to eliminate his breakfast meats altogether. I suggested that he try to replace some of the breakfast meat products with nuts. His wife placed a bowl of nuts on the breakfast table and began to serve smaller portions of the meat products. John was amazed that his new diet was not only not hard to eat, but so enjoyable that he did not crave those high-fat meats anymore!

NUT MILKS

Nut milks are not very commonly used in the United States, but they are so delicious, nutritious, and easy to digest that it is time you give them a try. We have seen that through the ages, people have made beverages out of nuts. They knew that tree nuts were well-balanced superfoods. Making them into milks made them easy to digest. All nuts can be used to make nut milks. A great use of nut milks is to pour them over your breakfast cereals.

Nut milks are coming back on the market: look for them with other specialty milks, like soy milk, in the refrigerated section of a good store, or look on the shelf for the kind that is packaged so that it remains fresh without refrigeration. You can also make your own nut milk at home: place about one ounce of nuts in a good blender with one or two cups of water, depending on how thick or thin you'd like your milk to be, and a natural sweetener of your choice, like honey, to taste. Blend well, and drink right away, or refrigerate for later use. For variety, use a fruit or vegetable juice instead of water and vary your sweetener, using maple syrup, brown sugar, or molasses instead of honey. Recipes for nut milks can be found in many books, including Candia Cole's *Not Milk . . . Nut Milks!*

In southern Italy, in Puglia, a province proud of its olives, nuts, and grains, a woman at a street stand sells prepared foods. The drink is almond milk. "Sometimes we make it [nut milk] with other nuts," she says, "like hazelnuts or pine nuts. People here love these nut milks." A mother and her child stop to refresh themselves with this balanced beverage with its protein, good energy, calcium, and all the other goodness of nuts. "I asked my grandmother once about nut milks," says the mother, "and she told me that her own grandmother had passed the recipe down and had told her that it was going back to centuries before she was born."

It's sad to see how nut milks have become such a rare food in our modern societies. Nut milks can be made from any tree nut, giving us variety of taste and valuable compounds.

NUTS AS APPETIZERS

Eating nuts as appetizers—hors d'oeuvres—is one of the uses of nuts that needs little introduction. A bowl of nuts, together with beverages or other foods before dinner, is a common way to serve nuts. But you can go beyond a simple bowl of nuts. You may roast your nuts (or buy them prepared) with herbs, bake some light nut wafers or biscuits or prepare some nut breads (see page 126 for more on nut breads). Another way is to serve some nut butter, made from your favorite nut, in a bowl on a tray with crackers and raw vegetables. To be fancy, offer more than one kind of nut butter. See page 125 for more on nut butters.

NUTS IN SALADS AND WITH VEGETABLES DISHES

Nut oils in salad dressing can add a nutty flavor to your favorite salad, and chopped nuts make a terrific addition to all green or mixed vegetable salads and fruit salads. Some of the smaller nuts, like pine nuts, can be used whole. Another way is to prepare a salad dressing by placing some nuts in a blender with your oil, vinegar, and salt. A classic salad that uses nuts is the Waldorf salad, created before the turn of the century by Oscar Tschirky, known as Oscar of the Waldorf, the maître d'hôtel at the old Waldorf-Astoria Hotel in New York City.

Chopped nuts also blend well with all kinds of cooked vegetables. Add some to your stir-fry or to a microwaved or oven-baked vegetable. You may add the nuts before cooking or just before serving the vegetables. Adding nuts to vegetable dishes makes them so flavorful that even people who tend not to eat enough vegetables find their nut-flavored vegetable dishes enjoyable, thus adding the nutritional benefits of nuts to those of the vegetables.

NUT SOUPS

The use of nuts in soups is a traditional one that parallels the use of nuts to make milk. The variety of possible soups is endless, and each nut can give a soup a unique flavor. The use of nuts in soups needs to make a major comeback. Not only is this a way to prepare delicious soups, but it is a major step toward making healthier soups, as the protein and fat of the nut can replace some or all of the protein and fat of meats or fowl. Either by making a meat and nut soup or by eliminating meats and fowl altogether from the soup and replacing them with nuts, you'll have made a much healthier soup.

Remember that adding nuts to a meat or chicken soup stock will make the balance of the fat much healthier by increasing the amount of unsaturated fat and decreasing that of the saturated fat.

A vegetable soup stock can be made with just nuts and vegetables. Grind the nuts in a food processor or blender, or chop them and use them raw or preroasted. Can you begin to see the tremendous variety you can have? Use herbs freely—for Mediterranean flavors, use sage, rosemary, thyme, oregano, or basil.

If one of your family members thinks he or she cannot cut down on meat, introduce nuts slowly into your soups, and watch his or her cholesterol go down! And your children will love your nut soups.

NUTS WITH PASTAS AND GRAINS

Not only do breakfast cereals profit by the addition of nuts, but adding nuts to pasta, rice, and other grain dishes is the perfect way to add great nutritional value and flavor. The protein and the balanced fats of the nut complement grains in a wonderful way. Pesto sauces—which can be made not only with pine nuts, but with other nuts as well—are one way to add nuts to pastas. You may sprinkle some ground or chopped nuts over your grain dish after cooking, or you can cook a grain, such as rice, in a broth that contains ground nuts.

Nuts added to grain dishes for lunch or dinner satisfy the desire for some fat.

NUTS WITH MEATS, POULTRY, AND FISH

Use nuts, chopped or ground, in all kinds of meats, poultry, and fish dishes. An easy way to use them in your cooking is to sprinkle nuts on fish, chicken, and meats before baking or grilling. Another way is to add nuts to poultry stuffing.

NUT PATTIES, BURGERS, AND LOAVES

Nut patties or nut burgers are becoming more and more popular. They are commonly found in supermarkets and are served by many restaurants, including fast-food restaurants. Ask for one of these for your next meal out. You can also try preparing nut burgers or nut loaves at home. They are generally prepared by grinding nuts and combining them with sautéed vegetables; precooked grains like rice, millet, barley, or wheat; soy products like tofu; and other ingredients of your choice. You may choose to use egg white as a binder. To make a burger, form into patties and gently grill or sauté in vegetable oil and serve as you would any meat; or shape it into a loaf and bake it. Consult almost any vegetarian cookbook for specifics on preparing a nut loaf or nut burger. If you are not ready to have a strictly vegetarian meal, you can add nuts to your meat-loaf for richer flavor and better nutrition.

NUT BUTTERS AND PASTES

Several different varieties of nut butters are available in many stores now. Or you can make your own in a food processor or proper blender following the manufacturer's instructions. Nut butters can be made from raw or roasted nuts. Mixing them with honey or other sweetener makes a delicious paste that you can spread on bread or just eat with a spoon. And you can use a nut paste to coat cakes for a delicious and healthy treat. Nut pastes are very popular in many countries.

NUT SAUCES

We learn from Claudia Roden, in her *A Book of Middle Eastern Food* that nuts have been used since ancient times in a variety of dishes and in unexpected ways. Each country has its own favorite way to prepare nuts. Egyptians or Syrians use ground almonds or pine nuts to thicken sauces, such as tarator, a sauce served over chicken, seafood, and vegetables, while in Turkey they use walnuts or hazelnuts. The faisinjan sauce for chicken or duck is made with nuts.

Mary Laird Hamady, in her book *Lebanese Mountain Cooking*, describes a fish sauce made with walnuts that often replaces the classic Lebanese tahini made with sesame seeds. Originally, this sauce was made by pounding the walnuts in a mortar, but you can make it in a blender. Other nuts can be used for variety.

Debbie Whittaker, editor of the *Herb Gourmet* newsletter, likes the combination of fresh herbs and nuts in pesto. She suggests making trendy versions of the traditional basil and pine nut Pesto Genovese, suggesting a blend of a wide variety of nuts and herbs, including hazelnuts, Brazil nuts, or walnuts with mint, lemon balm, or tarragon. The combinations are virtually endless. Originally, the Italians just pulverized fresh basil with olive oil with a mortar and pestle, but the recipes have evolved to include nuts and other herbs, along with garlic and Parmesan.

NUTS IN BREADS, PASTRIES, AND CAKES

In the Balkan States, people welcome the new walnut season by adding walnut pieces to their daily bread. The Middle Eastern flat bread Iflagun, described by Claudia Roden in *A Book of Middle Eastern Food* is covered with a spiced mixture of chopped pistachio nuts and a dry grating cheese. Other nuts can also be used for this bread. Was this the forerunner of pizza? In the Alpine region of Tyrol, they decorate the top of a simple long loaf with a line of hazelnuts, so that they roast gently during the baking of the bread. The Tyroleans also enrich savory whole-grain breads with finely ground almonds, hazelnuts, and pistachio nuts. Each country in Europe has a characteristic sweet Christmas bread made with the addition of a combination of nut pieces and dried fruits such as raisins; panettone from Italy and stollen from Germany are examples of European Christmas breads. Nut banana loaf is a delicious example of a dessert bread that combines nut pieces with fruit, in an otherwise simple quick bread. Any nut can be used to make delicious breads with unique flavors.

Danish pastries filled with almond paste and covered with chopped almonds or hazelnuts, are only examples of many nut-filled cakes and pastries from Scandinavia. They can be made with any tree nut. Pie crust for fruit pies and tarts can be shortened with finely ground nuts. Pie made from the native-American pecan is the classic of North American tables during the Thanksgiving holiday season. Pecans in their prime have wonderful maple flavor notes, so maple syrup is the ideal syrup to use in the pecan pie. This same style of pie could easily be made with walnuts, and then why not with almonds, cashews, hazelnuts, pine nuts, or any of the other tree nuts.

Dundee fruitcake from Scotland has chopped almonds in the cake and whole nuts decorating the top. A similar cake, topped with marzipan nut paste and icing, is the traditional Christmas and New Year's cake in Britain. A day-to-day dessert cake can be made with ground nuts taking the place of some flour. This cake needs no added fat or oil. Nut pieces can be added to dessert cakes, perhaps with some warming spice, such as cinnamon, or orange zest and juice.

NUTS IN COOKIES

Perhaps the most characteristic Italian biscotti are made with hazelnuts and almonds. The nuts are added whole to the dough, and during the second baking they gently roast. In Greece, a classic cookie is made simply from finely ground nuts, sugar, and flavored water, which is actually a nut paste. A cookie can be made just from finely ground nuts and honey, and could be flavored with rosewater. A similar cookie from Italy is an expansion of this delicious combination, made with egg whites, to produce the famous Amaretti or macaroons. Shortbread shortened with ground nuts is great as a delicious alternative to butter shortbread. Variations on nut paste cookies are to be found in all Scandinavian cookbooks. In Scandinavia, nut cookies are made for the Christmas holidays.

NUTS IN CANDIES AND BARS

Nougat made with pistachio, hazelnuts, and almonds; almond, Brazil-nut, pecan or hazelnut brittle; sugared almonds; honey almond chocolate bars; hazelnut-chocolate bars; pecan pralines; date and pecan rolls—these are just a few of the classic nut confections. Almond or hazelnut paste is a mixture of finely ground nuts and sugar with rose or orange water. It is used as the base for modeling miniature fruit and other designs for elegant and deliciously edible decorations, especially on celebration cakes. The combination gradually dries out, so there is usually no need to cook it.

On the market today are literally hundreds of snack bars made with dried fruits like raisins, nuts ground or whole, and other healthful ingredients. Try these during a break from athletic events, during a long hike, or during a break at the office: they satisfy and prevent the letdown that often comes after eating candies made with sugar alone.

NUTS IN FROZEN DESSERTS

Nuts are often found as additions to regular or low-fat ice cream. Frozen desserts can be made entirely from nut milks. If you choose to eat regular ice cream, which is fairly high in milk fat, the addition of nuts provides valuable unsaturated fats to the saturated fats of the milk. If the ice cream flavor you choose doesn't include nuts, you can chop some nuts and sprinkle them on top.

NUTS AS SNACKS AND SCHOOL LUNCHES

The nut and dried-fruit super snacks discussed in this chapter—nut bars, nuts alone or mixed with raisins and other dried fruits—are some of the healthiest snacks we can choose for adults and children. Take these snacks along to the office, to school, on a hike, or on a long drive. Encouraging children to eat this type of snack is crucial as it teaches them healthy eating habits. After reading this book, you can tell your child stories about the lore and romance of nuts to inspire them to eat nuts.

ROASTED NUTS

Roasting nuts in your home oven fills the kitchen with a unique nutty fragrance. Each nut has its own aroma, unique to the individual nut, from the scent of pines for pine nuts to the delicacy of hazelnuts and almonds. Roast nuts in an oven preheated to about 275 degrees Fahrenheit for 10 to 30 minutes.

NUT OILS

A little-known way to cut down on saturated fats is to replace dairy butter with a good oil. The Italians place some olive oil on a side dish for putting on bread, but a nut oil is another good choice. The French use almond, hazelnut, and walnut oils in addition to the classic olive oil. Remember that even the healthiest nut or olive oils should not be consumed in excess. Most fine food stores and natural food stores stock these oils.

SOME SUGGESTIONS FOR INCORPORATING NUTS INTO YOUR DIET FROM COOKBOOK AUTHORS

Lorna Sass, food historian and cookbook author, likes to eat Brazil nuts with dried apricots to add selenium to her diet, and she considers cardamom a great flavoring for nut dishes.

Paula Wolfert, author of *Mediterranean Grains and Greens* likes to use nuts to blend disparate flavors in sauces or other recipes. Fundamentally distinct or even contrasting flavors, like a pungent and a mild sweet one, are blended in a unique way by nuts.

Deborah Madison, author of *Vegetarian Cooking for Everyone*, likes to use roasted nuts or nuts freshly toasted in an ungreased skillet with salads. One of her cooked vegetable dishes combines Brussels sprouts, fennel, and pearl onions with walnuts. Other nuts can add variety to this dish.

Jesse Cool, chef and author, finds that nuts naturally lend themselves to preparing fall and winter dishes. "I use them roasted with cayenne and honey next to salads and hearty winter-greens; combine them with dried fruits; toss them with pastas and coat fish with crushed nuts. Blending nuts with savory grains and, of course, for desserts, nuts, fruit, and cheese are the perfect way to end a meal."

Monica Spiller, author of *The Barm Bakers' Book* and a researcher of whole-grain and ancient breads, likes to use nuts as part of naturally leavened whole-grain breads with some raisins added. She feels that ancient-style breads made with nuts and dried fruit are a wonderful way to add variety to meals.

Debbie Whittaker, food writer and editor of the *Herb Gourmet* newsletter, suggests purées of nuts, herbs, and oils to transform bland and simply prepared foods into gourmet fare. She likes to use nuts as a base for salad dressings, or stirred into white sauces, kneaded into breads, or just topped on steamed vegetables. She suggests tossing nuts with beans, rice, quinoa, or other grains; they create unusual side dishes.

REMEMBER VARIETY

Even though originally many classic recipes used the kind of nut that was native or easily available in that region, remember that most recipes can be made with just about any nut. This is important in our everyday life, as without some variety, we may get tired of even the greatest food. Choose different nuts and different ways to use them, and nuts will become an integral part of your diet, so that a day without nuts will seem strange to you.

Variety with the nuts we choose and the way we use them is a key to success. And not to be forgotten for the body-weight-conscious cook, adding nuts to a good diet will make your weight control easier, as you'll feel more satisfied after your meals or snacks.

Use the ideas from this chapter as a way to open the door to hundreds of recipes and uses of tree nuts. Thousands of pages would be needed to go into all the different uses and recipes for nuts. I have presented some basic suggestions to you as a starting point. Whether you are a creative cook, or you are just looking for simple ways to add nuts to your diet, the possibilities are endless.

Conclusion

As I began to work on this book—reading about all aspects of nuts, researching their history and science much more extensively than I had ever done before, and interviewing experts—something happened to me. Almost without realizing it, I wanted to eat more nuts, I wanted to eat nuts more often, and I wanted to eat a greater variety of nuts. I discovered that each nut has something special to offer. More frequently than ever, a bowl of nuts was on the table for breakfast, lunch, and dinner. When I had to go for a long drive, a bag of nuts and some raisins became my faithful companions. Nuts "grew" on me far beyond my expectations. What fascinated me was that I felt better and better as nuts became a more integral part of my way of life. I was feeling "superhealthy," and now I am a greater believer in nuts than ever before.

I have defined superfoods for you and explained why nuts are indeed superfoods that must be brought back to their proper place in our ways of life. The marvelous nutritional complexity of nuts, their good flavor, and the fact that they can be eaten raw with little preparation or in the most elaborate dishes prepared by a sophisticated chef should make it easy to bring nuts back into our ways of life. My own experience made me realize that there is more to the relationship of nuts to better health than a list of nutrients and well-known compounds. And it made me realize that the many myths and legends about nuts and their medicinal power had a lot of truth in them.

Base your diet on nuts, whole grains, beans, lentils, and plenty of fruits and vegetables. Add to this some reasonable amount of regular physical activity and you'll have made a major step in the prevention of major chronic disease. And you'll experience a new sense of wellness and joy of living. I hope this book will change forever the way you look at nuts and fats, as I know it will take time before some of the concepts in this book will be widely accepted by a society hit every day by low fat messages.

Now that you have read this book, shock your friends by telling them the science, the wonders, and the ancient history of nuts and the "good fats." Tell them the science, the lore, and the fascinating history of the little seeds from the precious nut trees of the world. You'll help them to better health.

And now, as I set aside this manuscript, I shall make myself a glass of fresh nut milk with a little honey and enjoy all of the goodness that nuts have to offer.

Glossary

Amino acids. The building blocks of proteins.

Antioxidant. A substance, such as vitamin E, selenium, and many other organic or inorganic compounds, capable of counteracting oxidative damage in animal and human tissue.

Arginine. An amino acid found in higher concentrations in nuts and other plant foods than in animal protein. It appears to have protective properties for the heart and arteries.

Atherosclerosis. Deposits in the arteries characterized by plaques containing cholesterol and lipids in the inner layers of the walls of some arteries.

Fiber. The part of plants and plant products consisting of complex carbohydrates and lignin that is not digestible by human digestive enzymes.

Folic acid. A B vitamin that makes the reproduction of cells, including blood cells, possible. It also lowers homocysteine levels in the blood, reducing the risk for heart disease. It is often low in American diets.

HDL (high-density lipoprotein). A globule that carries cholesterol in the blood. When cholesterol is in this form, it is considered to be protective and good, and is often called the "good cholesterol."

Homocysteine. An amino acid in the blood, high levels of which seem to indicate increased risk of heart disease.

Hydrogenated fats. Unsaturated fat treated with hydrogen under special chemical conditions to make them solid rather than liquid at room temperature. These are widely used in many prepared foods.

LDL (low-density lipoprotein). A globule that carries cholesterol in the blood. When cholesterol is in this form, it is considered to be much more damaging and to cause harmful deposits (plaques) in the arteries that slowly narrow the openings of the blood vessel. That's why it's often called the "bad cholesterol."

Lipoproteins. Globules in the blood composed of fats, proteins, and other compounds that carry cholesterol around in the blood. The two most commonly used in clinical medicine are the low-density lipoproteins (LDL) and high-density lipoproteins (HDL).

Monounsaturated fats. Fats with one double bond. When they replace saturated fats in the diet, they lower blood cholesterol. They are high in many nuts and olive oil.

Omega-3 fat. A special type of polyunsaturated fat that comes from fish and some plants.

Phytochemicals. Beneficial chemical compounds found in plant foods. *Phyto* means plant in Greek. Though these compounds are usually beneficial to health, they have not been considered important until recently.

Plant sterols. Compounds contained in plant foods that are somewhat similar in their chemical structure to cholesterol, but which actually help to lower blood cholesterol and may possibly have a protective effect against colon cancer.

Polyunsaturated fats. Fats with two or more double bonds. When they replace saturated fats in the diet, they lower blood cholesterol.

Unsaturated fats. Fats that have one or more double bonds between the carbon atoms in their molecules. This makes them more reactive than saturated fats. They are usually liquid at room temperature.

References

Many books and articles were consulted in the writing of this book. Those listed below were particularly helpful.

Abbey, M., et al. "Partial replacement of saturated fatty acids with almonds or walnuts lowers total plasma cholesterol and low-density-lipoprotein cholesterol." *American Journal of Clinical Nutrition* 59:995–999, 1994.

American Heart Association. *1998 Heart and Stroke Statistical Update.* American Heart Association, 1997.

Apicius, Gavius. *De Re Coquinaria (On Cooking).* edited and translated by Joseph Vehling. New York: Dover, 1977.

Berry, E., et al. "Effects of diets rich in monounsaturated fatty acids on plasma lipoproteins—the Jerusalem Nutrition Study: II. Monounsaturated fatty acids vs. carbohydrates." *American Journal of Clinical Nutrition* 56:394, 1992.

Berry, E., et al. Effects of diets rich in monounsaturated fatty acids on plasma lipoproteins—the Jerusalem Nutrition Study: high MUFAs vs. high PUFAS. *American Journal of Clinical Nutrition* 53:899, 1991.

Boorde, Andrew. *Dyetary.* F. J. Furnivall, ed. Early English Text Society, e.s. 10. London, 1870.

Bruce, B., G. A. Spiller, and J. W. Farquhar. "Effects of a plant-based diet rich in whole grains, sun-dried raisins and nuts on serum lipoproteins." *Vegetarian Nutrition: An International Journal* 1:58–63, 1997.

Coe, Sophie D. *America's First Cuisines*. Austin: University of Texas Press, 1994.

Cole, Candia Lea. *Not Milk . . . Nut Milks!* Santa Barbara, CA: Woodbridge Press, 1990.

Colquhoun, D., et al. "Comparison of a high monounsaturated fatty acid diet (enriched with macadamia nuts) and a high carbohydrate diet on blood lipids." Abstract presented at Proceedings of the 59TH European Atherosclerosis Congress, Nice, France, May, 1992.

Curb, J.D., et al. "Comparison of lipid levels in humans on a macadamia nut based high monounsaturated fat diet to their levels on a moderate fat diet and a high fat 'typical American' diet." Paper presented at the American Heart Association's Scientific Conference on Efficacy of Hypocholesterolemic Dietary Interventions, May 3–5, San Antonio, TX, 1995.

Darvill, Timothy. *Prehistoric Britain*. New Haven, CT: Yale University Press, 1987.

Dreher, M.L., C.V. Maher, and P. Kearney. "The traditional and emerging role of nuts in healthful diets." *Nutrition Reviews* 54: 241–245, 1996.

Farquhar, J.E. Plant sterols: their biological effects in humans. In Spiller, G., ed.: *Handbook of Lipids in Human Nutrition*. Boca Raton, FL: CRC Press, pp. 101–105, 1996.

Fraser, G.E., et al. "A possible protective effect of nut consumption on risk of coronary heart disease." *Archives of Internal Medicine* 152:1416–1424, 1992.

Gerspacher, Lucy. *Hazelnuts & More Cookbook*. Portland: Graphics Arts Center Publishing Company, 1995.

Hamady, Mary Laird. *Lebanese Mountain Cookery*. Boston: David R. Godine, Publisher, Inc., 1987.

Hartley, Dorothy. *Food in England*. London: Macdonald & Janes, 1954.

Heinerman, John. *Heinerman's Encyclopedia of Nuts, Berries and Seeds*. New York: Parker Publishing Company, 1995.

Hieatt, Constance B. and Butler, Sharon, ed. *Curye on Inglysch: English Culinary Manuscripts of the Fourteenth Century*. Toronto: Oxford University Press, 1985.

Ho, Chi-Tang, Chang Y. Lee, and Mou-Tuan Huang, eds. *Phenolic Compounds in Food and Their Effects on Health I*. Washington, D.C.: American Chemical Society, 1992.

Ho, Chi-Tang, et al., eds. *Food Phytochemicals for Cancer Prevention II*. Washington, D.C.: American Chemical Society, 1994.

Hora, Bayard, ed. *The Oxford Encyclopedia of Trees of the World*. New York: Crescent Books, 1980.

Hoshiyama, Y. and T. Sasaba. "A case-control study of single and multiple stomach cancers in Saitama Prefecture, Japan." *Japanese Journal of Cancer Research* 83:937–943, 1992.

Huang, Mou-Tuan, Chi-Tang Ho, and Chang Y. Lee, eds. *Phenolic Compounds in Food and Their Effects on Health II*. Washington, D.C.: American Chemical Society, 1992.

Johnson, Hugh. *The International Book of Trees*. New York: A. Gulf + Western Company, 1973.

Keys, A. *Seven Countries: A Multivariate Analysis of Death and Coronary Heart Disease*. Cambridge, MA: Harvard University Press, 1980.

Kitts, D. D. "Bioactive substances in food: identification and potential uses." *Canadian Journal of Physiological Pharmacy* 72:423–434, 1994.

Klevay, L. "Copper in nuts may lower heart disease risk." *Archives of Internal Medicine* 153:401–402, 1993.

Kritchevsky, D., et al. "Atherogenicity of animal and vegetable protein—influence of the lysine to arginine ratio. *Atherosclerosis* 41:429, 1982.

Lu, Henry C. *Chinese System of Food Cures.* New York: Sterling Publishing Co., Inc., 1986.

Madison, Deborah. *Vegetarian Cooking for Everyone.* New York: Broadway Books, 1997.

McCarrison, Sir Robert. *Studies in Deficiency Disease,* London: Henry Frowde and Hodder & Stoughton, 1921.

Menninger, Edwin A. *Edible Nuts of the World.* Stuart, FL: Horticultural Books, Inc., 1977.

Mensink, R.P. and M.B. Katan. "Effect of monounsaturated fatty acids versus complex carbohydrates on high density lipoproteins in healthy men and women." *Lancet* 1:122–125, 1987.

Mensink, R.P. and M.B. Katan. "Effect of a diet enriched with monounsaturated or polyunsaturated fatty acids on levels of low density and high density lipoprotein cholesterol in healthy women and men." *New England Journal of Medicine* 321:436–437, 1989.

Oakenfull, D. Saponins in the treatment of hypercholesterolemia. In Spiller, G.A., ed.: *Handbook of Lipids in Human Nutrition.* Boca Raton, FL: CRC Press, pp. 107–112, 1996.

Paul, A.A. and Southgate, D.A.T. *The Composition of Foods,* 4TH ed. London: Elsevier/North-Holland Biomedical Press, 1978.

Prineas, R.J., et al. "Walnuts and serum lipids." *New England Journal of Medicine* 359:329, 1993.

Reed, Mary. *Fruits & Nuts in Symbolism & Celebration.* San Jose, CA: Resource Publications, Inc., 1992.

Renfrew, Jane. *Food and Cooking in Prehistoric Britain, History and Recipes.* England: Historic Buildings and Monuments Commission, 1985.

Revel, Jean-François. *Culture & Cuisine.* New York: Doubleday & Co., Inc., 1982.

Roden, Claudia. *A Book of Middle Eastern Food.* New York: Vintage Books, 1974.

Sabaté, J., H.E.T. Bell, and G.E. Fraser. "Nut consumption and coronary heart disease risk." In Spiller, G.A., ed.: *Handbook of Lipids in Human Nutrition.* Boca Raton, FL: CRC Press, pp. 145–151, 1996.

Sabaté, J. and G.E. Fraser. "The probable role of nuts in preventing coronary heart disease." *Primary Care* 19:65–72, 1993.

Sabaté, J., et al. "Effects of walnuts on serum lipid levels and blood pressure in normal men." *New England Journal of Medicine* 328: 603–607, 1993.

Sabaté, J. and D.G. Hook. "Almonds, walnuts and serum lipids," in Spiller, G.A., ed., *Handbook of Lipids in Human Nutrition.* Boca Raton, FL: CRC Press, 1996, pp. 137–144.

Sass, Lorna J. *Lorna Sass' Complete Vegetarian Kitchen.* New York: Hearts Books, 1992.

Sass, Lorna J. *To The King's Taste.* New York: St. Martin's/Marek, 1975.

Shigeura, G.T. and H. Ooka. *Macadamia Nuts in Hawaii: History and Production.* Research Extension Series 039, 630 April, 1984.

Spiller, G.A., B. Bruce, and J.W. Farquhar. "Lipid-lowering effect of a Mediterranean-type diet high in total and soluble fiber and monounsaturated fat." *Circulation* 93:632, 1996.

Spiller, G.A., et al. "Diets high in phytochemicals and fiber may decrease the need for intrinsic defense against oxidative damage." Paper presented at the Experimental Biology 1997 Meetings of The American Physiological Society, New Orleans, LA, April 6–9 1997.

Spiller, G.A., et al. "Effect of two foods high in monounsaturated fat on plasma cholesterol and lipoproteins in adult humans." *American Journal of Clinical Nutrition* 51:524, 1990.

Spiller, G.A., et al. "Nuts and plasma lipids: an almond-based diet lowers LDL-C while preserving HDL-C." *Journal of the American College of Nutrition* 17:285–290, 1998.

Spiller, G.A., et al. "Effect of a diet high in monounsaturated fat from almonds on plasma cholesterol and lipoproteins." *Journal of the American College of Nutrition* 11:126–130, 1992.

Spiller, Gene A., ed. *The Mediterranean Diets in Health and Disease.* New York: Van Nostrand, 1991.

Spiller, Gene A., ed. *Dietary Fiber in Human Nutrition,* 2ND ed. Boca Raton, FL: CRC Press, 1993.

Spiller, Gene. *The Superpyramid Eating Program.* New York: Times Books, 1993.

Spiller, Gene A., ed. *Handbook of Lipids in Human Nutrition.* Boca Raton, FL: CRC Press, 1996.

Spiller, Gene and Rowena Hubbard. *Nutrition Secrets of the Ancients.* Rocklin, CA: Prima, 1996.

Spiller, Monica. *The Barm Bakers' Book.* Los Altos, CA: Sphera Press, 1992.

Tannahill, Reay. *Food in History.* New York: Stein and Day, 1973.

Tannahill, Reay. *Food in History.* New York: Crown Publishers, Inc., 1989.

The Visual Food Encyclopedia. Montreal: Québec/Amérique International, 1996.

Thoreau, Henry D. *Faith in a Seed.* Covelo, CA: Shearwater Books, 1993.

U. S. Department of Agriculture. *Composition of Foods: Nuts and Seed Products.* (Agricultural Handbook no. 8–12). Washington, DC: United States Department of Agriculture, 1984.

Vitale, Alice Thoms. *Leaves in Myth, Magic & Medicine.* New York: Stewart, Tabori & Chang, 1997.

Willan, Anne. *Great Cooks and Their Recipes: From Taillevent to Escoffier.* New York: Bullfinch Press, 1992.

Wills, Wirt H. *Early Prehistoric Agriculture in the American Southwest.* Santa Fe, NM: School of American Research Press, 1988.

Wolfert, Paula. *Mediterranean Grains and Greens.* New York: Harper Collins, 1998.

Woodroof, Jasper G. *Tree Nuts.* Westport, CT: AVI, 1979.

Sources of Information on Tree Nuts

The organizations that follow can supply you with nutritional and other information about tree nuts and their uses. In addition, these organizations support scientific research and education on the health benefits of tree nuts.

Almond Board of California
1104 12th Street
Modesto, CA 95354
Phone (209) 549–8262
Fax (209) 549–8267

Cashew Council
c/o Association of Food
   Industries
5 Ravine Drive
P.O. Box 545
Matawan, NJ 07747
Phone (732) 583–8188
Fax (732) 583–0798

Hazelnut Marketing Board
21595-A Dolores Way NE
Aurora, OR 97002
Phone (503) 678–6823
Fax (503) 678–6825

**International Tree Nut
   Council**
C/. Boule, 2
43201 Reus, Spain
Phone (34) 977–331416
Fax (34) 977–315028

MacFarms of Hawaii
89-406 Mamalohoa Highway
Captain Cook, HI 96704
Phone (808) 328–2435
Fax (808) 328–8081

**Santa Cruz Valley Pecan
Company**
1525 E. Helmut Peak Road
Sahuarita, AZ 85629
Phone (520) 791–2852
Fax (520) 791–2853

**California Pistachio
Commission**
1318 Shaw Avenue, Suite 420
Fresno, CA 93710
Phone (559) 221–8294
Fax (559) 221–8044

**California Walnut
Commission**
1540 River Park Drive,
Suite 101
Sacramento, CA 95815
Phone (916) 646–3807
Fax (916) 923–2548

**Health Research and Studies
Center and Sphera
Foundation**
P.O. Box 338
Los Altos, CA 94023–0338
Phone (650) 941–7251
Fax (650) 948–8540
Email: hrscenter@aol.com
Website: www.sphera.org

Index

Healthy Habits

are easy to come by—

IF YOU KNOW WHERE TO LOOK!

Get the latest information on:

- **better health • diet & weight loss**
- **the latest nutritional supplements**
- **herbal healing • homeopathy and more**

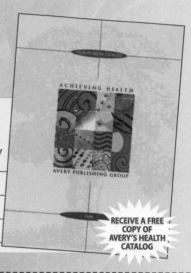

COMPLETE AND RETURN THIS CARD RIGHT AWAY!

Where did you purchase this book?

- ❑ bookstore
- ❑ supermarket
- ❑ health food store
- ❑ other (please specify)_____
- ❑ pharmacy

Name_____

Street Address_____

City_____State_____Zip_____

RECEIVE A FREE COPY OF AVERY'S HEALTH CATALOG

GIVE ONE TO A FRIEND ...

Healthy Habits

are easy to come by—

IF YOU KNOW WHERE TO LOOK!

Get the latest information on:

- **better health • diet & weight loss**
- **the latest nutritional supplements**
- **herbal healing • homeopathy and more**

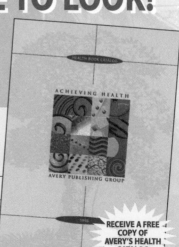

COMPLETE AND RETURN THIS CARD RIGHT AWAY!

Where did you purchase this book?

- ❑ bookstore
- ❑ supermarket
- ❑ health food store
- ❑ other (please specify)_____
- ❑ pharmacy

Name_____

Street Address_____

City_____State_____Zip_____

RECEIVE A FREE COPY OF AVERY'S HEALTH CATALOG

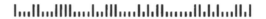